EDS Official Organ of European Digestive Surgery

Digestive Surgery

KARGER

Printed in Switzerland
on acid-free paper by
Thür AG Offsetdruck, Pratteln

Appears bimonthly:
1 volume per year (6 issues)

Digestive Surgery

Submission: Only original papers written in English are considered and should be sent to:

Prof. Dr. M.W. Büchler
Klinik für Viszerale und
Transplantationschirurgie
Inselspital Bern
CH–3010 Bern (Switzerland)

or

Prof. Dr. E.H. Farthmann
Chirurgische Universitätsklinik
Hugstetter Strasse 55
D–79106 Freiburg (Germany)

Manuscripts should be submitted in quadruplicate (with four sets of illustrations of which one is an original), typewritten double-spaced on one side of the paper, with a wide margin.

Conditions: All manuscripts are subject to editorial review. Manuscripts are received with the explicit understanding that they are not under simultaneous consideration by any other publication. Submission of an article for publication implies the transfer of the copyright from the author to the publisher upon acceptance. Accepted papers become the permanent property of 'Digestive Surgery' and may not be reproduced by any means, in whole or in part, without the written consent of the publisher. It is the author's responsibility to obtain permission to reproduce illustrations, tables, etc. from other publications.
The journal consists of the following sections:
1. Editorials
2. Review Articles
3. Original Papers
* 4. How I do it
5. Case Reports
6. Announcements

Arrangement

Title page: The first page of each paper should indicate the title (main title underlined), the authors' names, and the institute where the work was conducted. A short title for use as running head as well as the full address of the author to whom correspondence should be sent are also required.

Full address: The exact postal address complete with postal code must be given at the bottom of the title page. Please also supply Phone, Fax, and E-mail numbers.

Key words: For indexing purposes, a list of 3–10 key words in English is essential.

Abstract: Each paper needs an abstract of up to 10 lines.

Small type: Paragraphs which can or must be set in smaller type (case histories, test methods, etc.) should be indicated with a 'p' (petit) in the margin on the left-hand side.

Footnotes: Avoid footnotes. When essential, they are numbered consecutively and typed at the foot of the appropriate page.

Tables and illustrations: Tables and illustrations (both numbered in Arabic numerals) should be prepared on separate sheets. Tables require a heading and figures a legend, also prepared on a separate sheet. For the reproduction of illustrations, good drawings and original photographs are preferred; slides may also be accepted; negatives or photocopies cannot be used. Due to technical reasons, figures with a screen background should not be submitted. When possible, group several illustrations on one block for reproduction (max. size 181 × 223 mm) or provide crop marks. On the back of each illustration, indicate its number, the author's name, and 'top' with a soft pencil.

Color illustrations: Up to 6 color illustrations per page can now be integrated with the text at the reduced price of CHF 600.–/USD 545.00 per page. Color illustrations are reproduced at the author's expense.

References: In the text identify references by Arabic numerals [in square brackets]. Material submitted for publication but not yet accepted should be noted as 'unpublished data' and not be included in the reference list. The list of references should include only those publications which are cited in the text. Do not alphabetize; number references in the order in which they are first mentioned in the text. The surnames of the authors followed by initials should be given. There should be no punctuation other than a comma to separate the authors. Cite all authors, 'et al' is not sufficient. Abbreviate journal names according to the Index Medicus system. (Also see International Committee of Medical Journal Editors: Uniform requirements for manuscripts submitted to biomedical journals. Br Med J 1988;296:401–405.)
Examples
(a) Papers published in periodicals: Kauffman HF, van der Heide S, Beaumont F, Blok H, de Vries K: Class-specific antibody determination against *Aspergillus fumigatus* by means of the enzyme-linked immunosorbent assay. III. Comparative study: IgG, IgA, IgM ELISA titers, precipitating antibodies and IgE binding after fractionation of the antigen. Int Arch Allergy Appl Immunol 1986;80:300–306.
(b) Monographs: Matthews DE, Farewell VT: Using and Understanding Medical Statistics. Basel, Karger, 1985.
(c) Edited books: Hardy WD Jr, Essex M: FeLV-induced feline acquired immune deficiency syndrome: A model for human AIDS; in Klein E (ed): Acquired Immunodeficiency Syndrome. Prog Allergy. Basel, Karger, 1986, vol 37, pp 353–376.
Further details: Authors may consult our leaflet 'Rules for the Preparation of Manuscripts', available on request from the Publisher, S. Karger AG, P.O. Box, CH–4009 Basel (Switzerland).

Galley proofs: Unless indicated otherwise, galley proofs are sent to the first-named author and should be returned with the least possible delay. Alterations made in galley proofs, other than the correction of printer's errors, are charged to the author. No page proofs are supplied.

Reprints: Order forms and a price list are sent with the galley proofs. Orders submitted after the issue is printed are subject to considerably higher prices. Allow five weeks from date of publication for delivery of reprints.

* How I do it

Digestive Surgery is publishing articles which describe modern operative techniques in the field of Gastrointestinal Surgery.
The manuscript should be short and precise (maximum 10 typewritten double spaced pages) and should contain 1–4 figures to explain the surgical procedure.
Decisions of submitted papers within 6 weeks: A decision will be reached within 6 weeks for manuscripts submitted to the 'How I do it' section.

General Information

Digestive Surgery

Publication data: 'Digestive Surgery' is published 6 times annually. Volume 12 with 6 issues appears in 1995.

Subscription rates: Subscriptions run for a full calendar year. Prices are given per volume.

Personal subscription:

Subscription	*+ postage and handling*	
SFr. 313.50	+ SFr. 12.80	Europe
SFr. 313.50	+ SFr. 19.50	Overseas
US$ 241.00	+ US$ 12.80	

(Must be in the name of, billed to, and paid by an individual. Order must be marked 'personal subscription'.)

Institutional subscription:

Subscription	*+ postage and handling*	
SFr. 627.–	+ SFr. 25.50	Europe
SFr. 627.–	+ SFr. 39.–	Overseas
US$ 482.00	+ US$ 25.50	

Airmail postage: SFr. 36.–, US$ 30.00. (Extra per volume.)

Microforms: Please direct all enquiries and orders to:
University Microfilms Inc.
300 North Zeeb Road, P.O. Box 1346
Ann Arbor, MI 48106-1346 (USA)

Subscription orders: Orders can be placed at agencies, bookstores, directly with the Publisher S. Karger AG, P.O. Box, CH – 4009 Basel (Switzerland) or with any of the following distributors:

Deutschland: S. Karger GmbH, Postfach
D – 79095 Freiburg

France: Librairie Luginbühl
36, bd de Latour-Maubourg, F–75007 Paris

Great Britain, Ireland: S. Karger Publishers
11 Ravenscroft Road
Beckenham, Kent BR3 4TP

USA: S. Karger Publishers, Inc.
26 West Avon Road, P.O. Box 529
Farmington, CT 06085

India, Bangladesh, Sri Lanka:
S. Karger India Subscription Agency
B – 5/132 Safdarjung Enclave
New Delhi-110029

Japan: Katakura Libri, Inc.
Take 1 Bldg, 2nd Floor, 4-5-7 Yushima
Bunkyo-ku, Tokyo 113

Change of address: Both old and new address should be sent to the subscription source.

Single issues and back volumes: Information can be obtained through the Publisher.

Advertising: Correspondence and rate requests should be addressed to the Publisher.

Bibliographic indices: This journal is regularly listed in bibliographic services.

Book Reviews: Books are accepted for review by special agreement.

KARGER

Laparoscopic Colorectal Surgery

Editors
M.W. Büchler, Bern
L. Krähenbühl, Bern

18 figures, 36 tables, 1996

KARGER

S. Karger
Medical and Scientific Publishers
Basel · Freiburg · Paris · London
New York · New Delhi · Bangkok
Singapore · Tokyo · Sydney

Drug Dosage
The authors and the publisher have exerted every effort to ensure that drug selection and dosage set forth in this text are in accord with current recommendations and practice at the time of publication. However, in view of ongoing research, changes in government regulations, and the constant flow of information relating to drug therapy and drug reactions, the reader is urged to check the package insert for each drug for any change in indications and dosage and for added warnings and precautions. This is particularly important when the recommended agent is a new and/or infrequently employed drug.

Printed in Switzerland on acid-free paper by
Thür AG Offsetdruck, Pratteln
ISBN 3–8055–6282–9

Contents

Editorial

Dig Surg 1995;12:269–270

L. Krähenbühl
M.W. Büchler

Visceral and Transplantation Surgery, University of Berne, Inselspital, Berne, Switzerland

Laparoscopic Colon Surgery: Do We Need It?

When the first laparoscopic cholecystectomy was performed, a new revolution in general surgery began, and other abdominal surgical procedures such as appendectomy, hernia repair and fundoplication were given access to minimal invasive surgery. The main conclusion from our second international laparoscopic meeting (Five Years of Laparoscopic Cholecystectomy: A Reappraisal, Berne, 5–6 May 1995) was that laparoscopic cholecystectomy is now the standard treatment for symptomatic gallstone disease; and even for acute cholecystitis this approach seems to be the procedure of choice [1]. The advantages of laparoscopy over conventional open surgery are less postoperative pain, shorter hospital stay, less absence from work, less postoperative morbidity, fewer adhesions with less frequent postoperative bowel obstruction, superior cosmetic results, and, as shown in recent studies, diminished postoperative stress response due to the reduced abdominal wall trauma. The first case report for laparoscopic assisted sigmoid resection was published in June 1991 [2], and the first larger series with 20 resections (12 for malignancies) was published in the same 1991 issue by Jacobs et al. [3]. They showed that laparoscopically assisted colon surgery was feasible with less postoperative pain and a shortened hospital stay due to the diminished length of postoperative ileus and without any morbidity and mortality. By the following year, it was possible to perform almost every procedure in colorectal surgery laparoscopically; however, many serious or even life-threatening complications arose during the learning curve, such as major bleeding, bowel perforation, ureter and bladder injuries and cardiac and pulmonary problems due to the increased operating time with CO_2 pneumoperitoneum and the increased need for repeat operations [4]. Few authors have performed cost analyses, and the great majority of those who have, have not shown any significant advantages of the laparoscopic treatment [5]. Nevertheless, despite the absence of any prospective randomized clinical trials proving the superiority, or even the equivalence of laparoscopic colectomy compared with traditional open surgery, the new technique continued to be performed. When Alexander et al. [6] reported the first port side recurrence 3 months after an attempted curative laparoscopic assisted right hemicolectomy for a Duke's C adenocarcinoma, it became evident that laparoscopic colectomy for malignant disease should be approached with caution. At least 30 port side recurrences have now been reported in the literature [7]. This phenomenon causes concern for many reasons, including:

(1) Not all recurrences have been at the port through which the specimen was retrieved.

(2) The total actual number of recurrences and their incidence is unknown because there is a delay after their occurrence and also not all cases are published.

(3) Trocar metastases are not exclusive to advanced malignant disease. Today most of the reported cases have occurred after resection of Duke's B and C lesions, but at least 3 reports document trocar metastases for Duke's A lesions after curative laparoscopic colectomy [7].

(4) Wound recurrence is also a well-known problem following a standard laparotomy in colorectal surgery. Its estimated incidence is 1%, mainly for Duke's C and D lesions [8]. Throughout the published laparoscopic data its incidence is estimated at between 4 and 6% [7].

M.W. Büchler, MD
Visceral and Transplantation Surgery
University of Berne
Inselspital
CH–3010 Berne (Switzerland)

0253–4886/95/0125–0269
$ 8.00/0

The aims of colorectal cancer surgery are to improve the long-term cure, to reduce local recurrence rate and to improve overall quality of life. Until now, there has been no prospective randomized clinical trial available which compares open and laparoscopic techniques for this particular outcome, and long-term follow-up for laparoscopically treated malignant disease is unavailable. In our opinion, it is essential that only valid scientific data with long-term follow-up, and not the personal opinions of skilled laparoscopic teams, are needed to answer the question about which technique will best cure our patients of colorectal malignancy. Patients must not be sacrified to achieve triumph over technology.

Therefore, we strongly recommend that laparoscopic colon surgery for *malignant disease* should only be performed in randomized multicentre clinical trials. In contrast, however, laparoscopy might be a method for *benign disease* such as diverticulosis, Crohn's disease, ulcerative colitis, volvulus or rectum prolapse. Again, clinical trials must prove that the laparoscopic approach for benign colonic lesions provides advantages but these surgical procedures might be applied outside controlled clinical trials in specialized centres.

This issue of *Digestive Surgery* contains the manuscripts of an international workshop which took place at the university of Berne in May 1995.

References

1 Büchler MW, Frei E, Klaiber CH, Krähenbühl L: Five years of laparoscopic cholecystectomy: A reappraisal. Prog Surg. Basel, Karger (1996), in press.

2 Fowler DL, White SA: Laparoscopy-assisted sigmoid resection. Surg Laparosc Endosc 1991;1:183–188.

3 Jacobs M, Verdeja JC, Goldstein HS: Minimally invasive colon resection (laparoscopic colectomy). Surg Laparosc Endosc 1991;1:138–143.

4 Dean PA, Beart RW, Nelson H, Elftmann TD, Schlinkert RT: Laparoscopic-assisted segmental colectomy: Early Mayo Clinic experience. Mayo Clin Proc 1994;69:834–840.

5 Falk PM, Beart RW, Wexner SD, Thorson AG, Jagelman DG, et al: Laparoscopic colectomy: A critical appraisal. Dis Colon Rectum 1993;36:28–34.

6 Alexander RJT, Jaques BC, Mitchell KG: Laparoscopically assisted colectomy and wound recurrence. Lancet 1993;341:249–250.

7 Wexner SD, Cohen SM: Port site metastases after laparoscopic colorectal surgery for cure of malignancy. Br J Surg 1995;82:295–298.

8 Hughes ESR, McDermot FT, Polglase AL, Johnson WR: Tumor recurrence in the abdominal wall scar tissue after large-bowel cancer surgery. Dis Colon Rectum 1983;26:571–572.

Dig Surg 1995;12:271–276

Laparoscopic Colorectal Surgery

P. Petropoulos[a]
P. Kiesler[a]
Chr. Chanson[a]
K. Nassiopoulos[a]
R. Steffen[b]

[a] Department of General Surgery, Hôpital Cantonal Fribourg, and
[b] Clinique Beau-Site Bern, Switzerland

Key Words
Laparoscopic surgery · Diverticulitis · Sigmoidovesical fistulae · Colonic cancer

Introduction

Laparoscopic colorectal surgery (LCS) was first introduced in 1990 in the United States [1, 2]. The technique is still controversial and it is not yet widely used. Especially in cancer patients, an alarming number of port site metastasis has been reported [3–5]. However, with constantly improving instruments and optical equipment, LSC is applied with increasing frequency worldwide, more often in benign diseases.

Our group (table 1), consisting of 11 institutions, started LCS in October 1993, initially for benign diseases. Later, we enlarged our indications for malignant degenerated polyps, carcinomas in the rectosigmoid area smaller than 2 cm, carcinomas requiring rectal amputation, and tumors that already present with metastases.

In our view, it is important that a new technique should not, without good reason, change the principles of an already established surgical intervention. It is our policy to respect and adhere to the rules of open colorectal surgery which means clean operation fields, guarantee of blood supply, tension-free anastomosis, and radical excision. Increasing costs and demands on resources have to be considered as well.

Table 1. Associated institutions and number of operated patients

Institution			Patients n
Fribourg	Petropoulos	and hospital team	64
Aarau	Petropoulos	W. Zimmerli/ R. Hoffmann	2
Baden	Petropoulos	H. Säuberli	6
Bern (Clinique Beau Site)	Petropoulos	R. Steffen	15
Genève (HCUG)	Petropoulos	P. Ambrosetti	1
Lugano (Ospedale Regionale)	Petropoulos	R. von Huben	1
Montreux	Petropoulos	R. Cavin	18
Morges	Petropoulos	A. Meyer	6
Payerne	Petropoulos	O. Rostan	3
Vevey	Petropoulos	B. Cosandey	6
Yverdon	Petropoulos	J.F. Schmid	9
Total			131

Patients and Methods

From October 20, 1993 to April 30, 1995 our group performed 131 laparoscopic colorectal procedures. There were 56 females with a mean age of 64.4 years and 75 males with a mean age of 61.3 years.

Dr. P. Petropoulos
Médecin-chef, clinique de chirurgie générale
Hôpital Cantonal Fribourg
CH–1708 Fribourg (Switzerland)

0253–4886/95/0125–0271
$ 8.00/0

Table 2. Indications

Disease	Patients n
Crohn's disease of terminal ileum	1
Right colon polyps	3
Left colon polyps	6
Dolichocolon	2
Rectal prolapse	2
Diverticulitis of the sigmoid	77
Diverticulitis with sigmoidovesical fistulae	4
Sigmoid trauma	1
Right colon carcinoma	2
Malignant polyps of the left colon	3
Sigmoid carcinoma < 2 cm	13
Rectal carcinoma	17
Total	131

Table 3. Procedures

	Patients n
Ileocecal resection	1
Right hemicolectomy	5
Left hemicolectomy	5
Sigmoidectomy	92
Low anterior resection	15
Abdominoperineal resection	12
Bowel suture	1
Total	131

Ninety-six patients suffered from benign and 35 from malignant diseases (table 2). The various operations performed are listed in table 3.

Our technique for sigmoid resection is as follows:

Position of the Patient (fig. 1)
The patient is placed in a supine position with legs spread, the right leg a little lower than the left. The buttocks protrude over the lower edge of the operating table by about 10 cm to make subsequent stapler manipulations easier. The left buttock is slightly elevated and the patient is strapped well to the table to allow for a steep Trendelenburg position. Armrests above the patient's chest are for the surgeon and his assistants.

Team Position (fig. 2)
The surgeon stands to the right of the patient, to his left is the first assistant and the second assistant stands between the patient's legs. The instrument nurse and the instrument tables are placed between the surgeon and the second assistant. The team of anesthesists is, as usual, near the head of the patient.

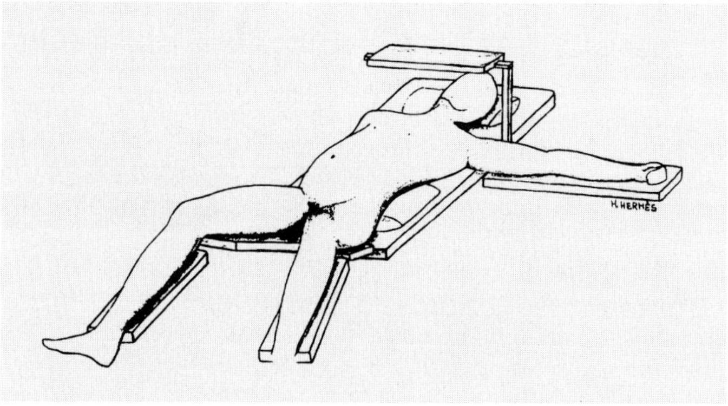

Fig. 1. Sigmoid resection: patient's position.

Position of the Video Column (fig. 2)
The video column is placed at the left near the feet of the patient. A second monitor may be placed at the left near the head.

Trocars Positioning (fig. 3)
Trocars are inserted in a circlewise position with the center of the circle in the left suprapubic region. We use a total of five trocars, two 10-mm trocars, two 10- to 12-mm trocars, and one 5-mm trocar.

Operation Technique
After creation of the CO_2 pneumoperitoneum to a pressure of 10–12 mm Hg, the trocars are placed as shown in figure 3.

First the coloparietal adhesions are incised (fig. 4) and the left colon is mobilised medially until the left ureter is identified. Mobilisation is continued up to the splenic flexure and down to the pelvis till the rectosigmoid junction and even lower.

The already mobilised part of the colon is now elevated laterally and the peritoneum of mesocolon is incised. The next step is identification of the proximal resection line. This should allow a tension-free anastomosis even if we have to extend down to the extraperitoneal rectal stump. An Endobabcock which gently grasps the hypothetical resection line is inserted through the left suprapubic trocar. The bowel is now pulled towards the trocar. If it reaches without any tension, the grasped region corresponds to the proximal resection line. Otherwise, a more distal resection line should be tried. An alternative could be further proximal mobilisation of the colon.

Now the mesocolon vessels corresponding to the segment that has to be resected are clipped or ligated and divided (fig. 5–8). The distal resection line is also prepared in the same way. The Endo-GIA is introduced from the right side and the colon is transected distally. The left suprapubic trocar wound is enlarged to a 4- to 6-cm minilaparotomy and the prepared segment of the colon is exteriorised (fig. 9), and proximally divided. Pneumoperitoneum is now inactive and that part of the operation is performed by classic surgery.

0.5-mg glucagon or 1 Amp. Buscopan is given intravenously by the anesthesist to help dilate the colon. A purse string with Prolen 2.0 is carried out and an appropriate circular stapler head is introduced to the lumen of descending colon and the purse string is tightened (fig. 10). The colon is then replaced into the abdominal cavity and the minilaparotomy is closed in layers; the closure should be airtight.

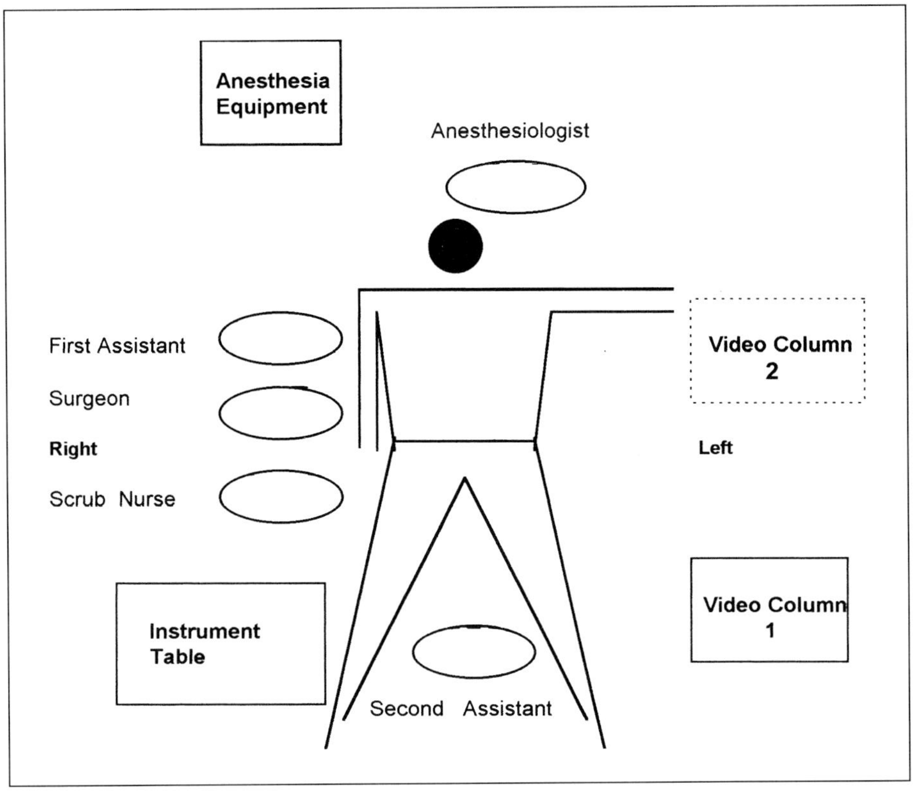

Fig. 2. Sigmoid resection: position of team and instruments.

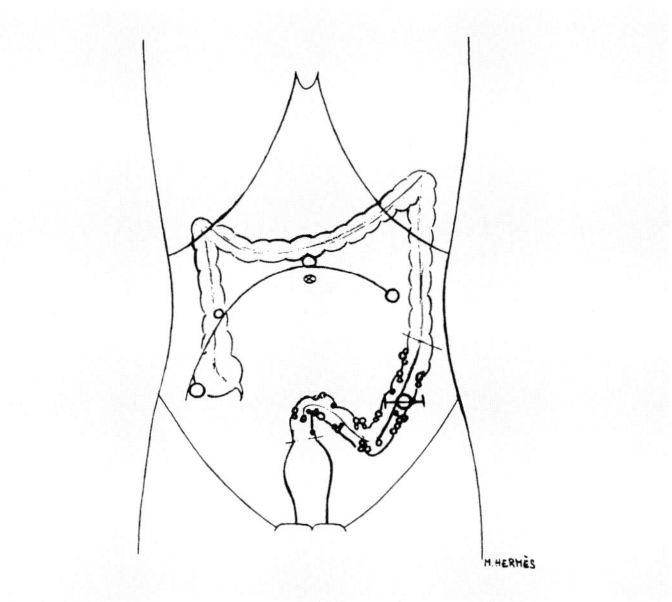

Fig. 3. Trocar placement for sigmoid resection.

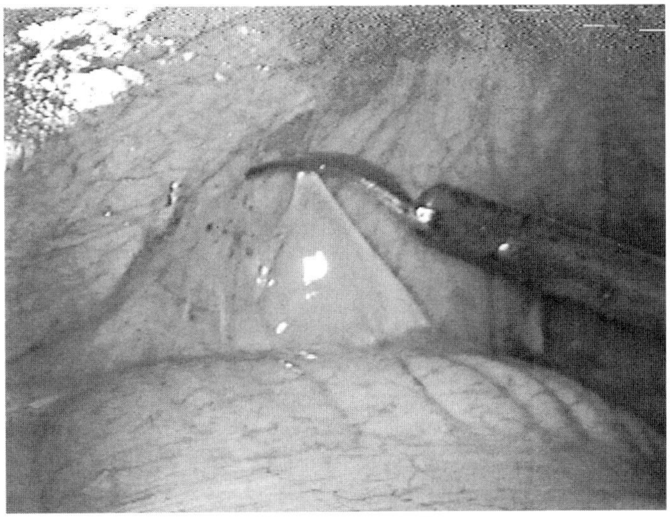

Fig. 4. Incision of coloparietal adhesions.

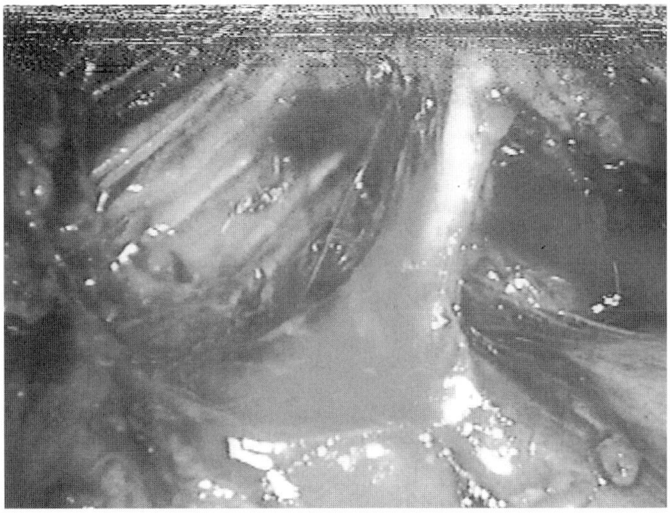

Fig. 5. Prepared inferior mesenteric artery.

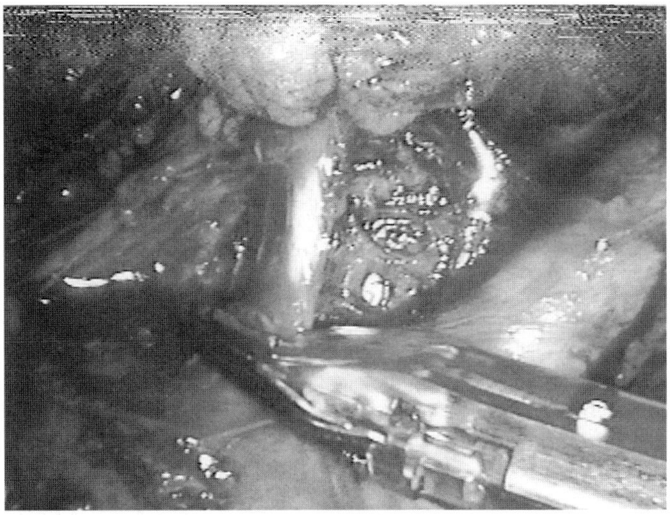

Fig. 6. Clipping of the inferior mesenteric artery.

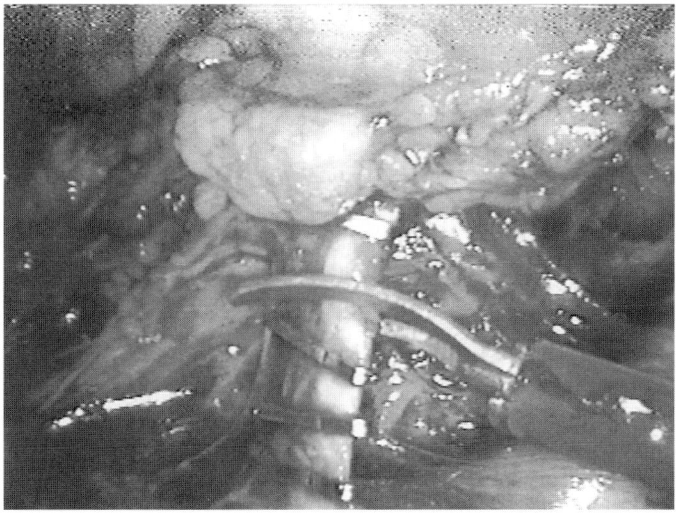

Fig. 7. Section of the clipped inferior mesenteric artery.

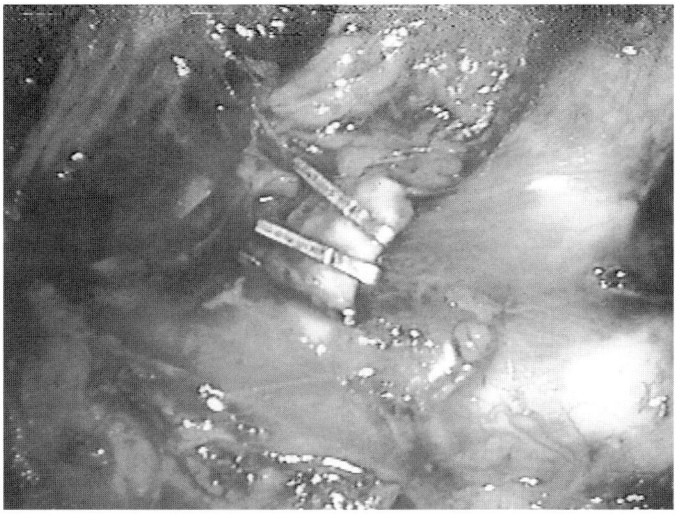

Fig. 8. Sectioned inferior mesenteric artery.

The pneumoperitoneum is recreated, the anal canal is gradually dilated and the circular stapler introduced. The head of the stapler is connected with the incorporated trocar at the main device and the anastomosis is performed under laparoscopic control (fig. 11).

The integrity of the anastomosis is now tested. The bowel is clamped proximal to the anastomosis with special forceps inserted through the trocar in the right iliac fossa. The Douglas is filled with physiologic saline and air is introduced into the rectum through a soft rectal catheter. These maneuvers are done under exact continuous laparoscopic control (fig. 12).

In case of sites of leakage, interrupted laparoscopic sutures can be placed. Drainage of this region is carried out only if the anastomosis does not seem to be fully closed and, of course, if the responsible surgeon finds it necessary. At the end of the operation, the pneumoperitoneum is released, the instruments are removed and closure of the wounds is undertaken.

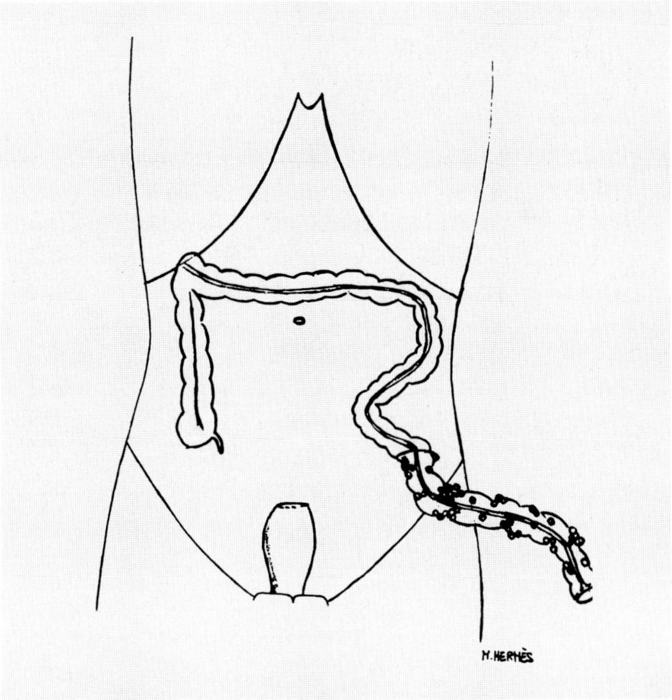

Fig. 9. Exteriorisation of prepared colon segment.

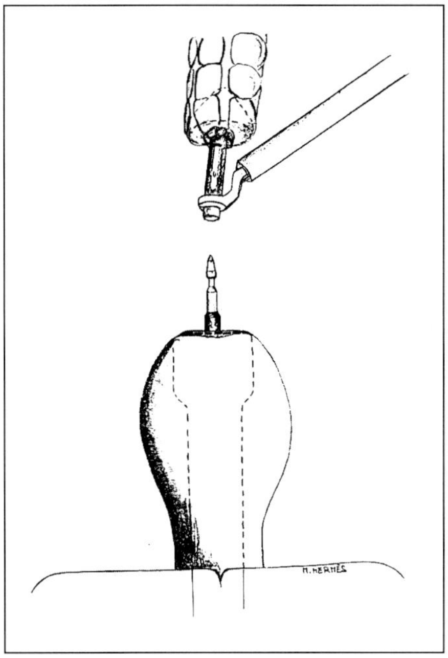

Fig. 10. Introduction of stapler head in the lumen of the discending colon.

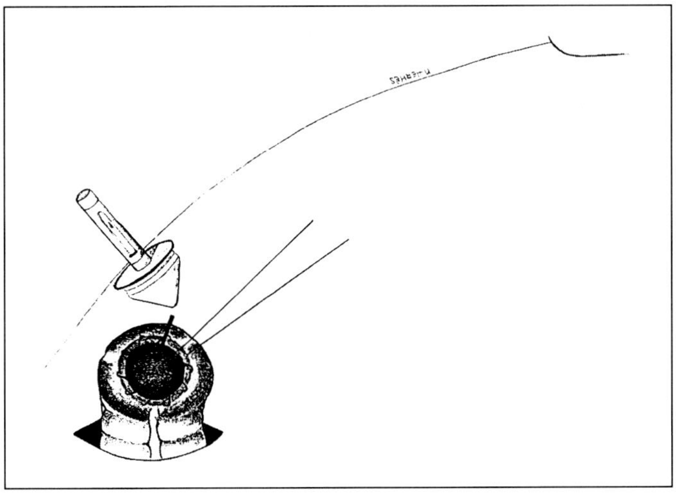

Fig. 11. Connection of the stapler head with the trocar of the main device.

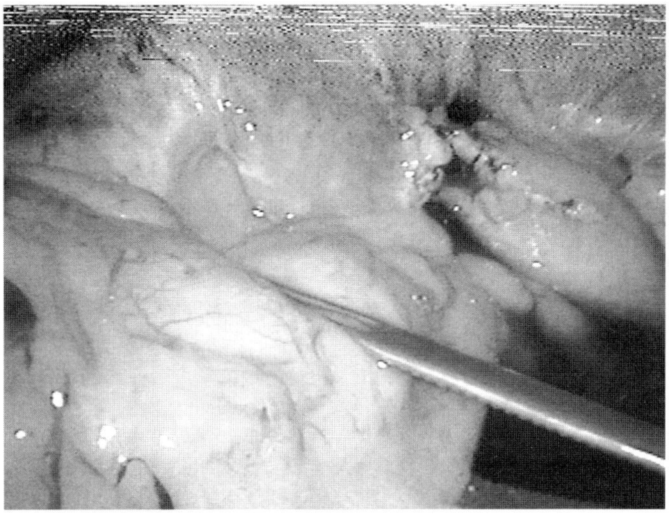

Fig. 12. Control of anastomosis integrity

Results

Of the 131 patients operated from October 20, 1993 through April 30, 1995, conversion had to be carried out 11 times (8.3%); the reasons for this conversion are listed in table 4.

Mean operative time was 1/3 longer than for a comparable open resection (table 5).

It is surprising how rapidly the patients recover after these operations with an especially rapid recovery of bowel function. A full oral intake can be initiated at the second postoperative day. Length of hospital stay as well as return

Table 4. Conversion (8.3%)

Reason	Patients n
Problem with aspiration	1
Problem with instruments	2
Inability to pass the stapler through the rectum	3
Diverticulitis abscess	1
Cancer extended to the uterus	1
Traumatism (iatrogenic) of the left ureter	1
Traumatism of the transversum with trocars	1
Rectal traumatism (iatrogenic)	1
Total	11

Table 5. Duration of operation

Procedures	Time h (range)
Right hemicolectomy	3.45 (3.0–4.30)
Left hemicolectomy	3.30 (3.0–4.0)
Sigmoidectomy	3.0 (1.15–5.0)
Low anterior resection	3.30 (2.10–5.0)
Abdominoperineal resection	4.15 (3.30–5.0)

to work is much shorter in comparison with conventional surgery. Postoperative complications and mortality are higher in patients with carcinoma than with benign diseases. Table 6 shows the observed complications and mortality. To now, we have not noticed any recurrence or metastases at the port sites in our 35 patients with tumors.

Table 6. Morbidity and mortality

		Patients n
Morbidity		
Seroma		1
Hematoma		4
Abdominal wall abscess		1
Anastomotic leak	→ conservative	2
Bleeding the 5th postop. day	→ laparotomy	1
Ileus with anastomotic leak	→ laparotomy	2
Stricture af the anastomosis	→ laparotomy	1
Bladder disorders		1
Total		13 (10%)
Mortality		
Septic shock (by malignancy)		1
Heart failure (by malignancy)		1
Total		2 (1.5%)

Conclusions

A laparoscopic approach for colon resection cannot be indicated generally. We are now fully convinced that this technique is the method of choice for benign diseases of the colon. The surgeons' training is of prime importance. This is more difficult to achieve in Switzerland with its limited number of patients. The answer might be laboratory work first and then tutoring and cooperation. As far as the latter is concerned, our group works closely together, sharing experience and knowledge. We are open for further cooperation.

It is very important for us to strictly control our cancer patients in order to observe recurrence or port site metastasis.

We are confident that laparoscopic colorectoral surgery will find its place in the treatment of large bowel diseases under conditions of good surgical education and appropriate indications.

References

1 Fowler DL, White SA: Laparoscopy-assisted sigmoid resection. Surg Laparosc Endosc 1991;1:183–188.
2 Jacob M, Verdeja JC, Goldstein HS: Minimally invasive colon resection (laparoscopic colectomy). Surg Laparosc Endosc 1991;1: 144–150.
3 Walsh DC, Wattchow DA: Subcutaneous metastases after laparoscopic resection of malignancy. Aust NZ J Surg 1993;63:563–565.
4 Wade TP, Comitalo JB, Andrus CH, Goodwin MN, Kaminski DL: Laparoscopic cancer surgery: Lessons from gallbladder cancer. Surg Endosc 1994;8:698–701.
5 Wexner SD, Cohen MS: Port site metastases after laparoscopic colorectal surgery for cure of malignancy. Br J Surg 1995;82:295–298.

Dig Surg 1996;12:277–279

Peter M.N.Y.H. Go

Department of Surgery,
St. Antonius Hospital, Nieuwegein,
The Netherlands

Laparoscopic Large Bowel Procedures

Key Words
Laparoscopic large bowel procedures · Port-site metastasis · Laparoscopic ultrasonic dissector · Laparoscopic ultrasonography

Introduction

In July 1991, Jansen performed the first laparoscopic large bowel procedure in The Netherlands. Subsequently, several laparoscopic pioneers start to perform these procedures. At the same time a debate started about the possible advantages of laparoscopic bowel resections. Laparoscopic bowel resections are time consuming, require much experience in laparoscopic surgery and are expensive for the usage of disposable instruments. In addition, the benefit of the laparoscopic operation to the patient is not so obvious as with laparoscopic cholecystectomy. There was also a concern how to keep up with oncologic principles as compared to conventional resections by laparotomy. The diffusion of laparoscopic bowel operations in The Netherlands is therefore rather slow, especially as compared to laparoscopic cholecystectomy. In June 1994, a national survey indicated that laparoscopic cholecystectomy was being performed in all Dutch hospitals, but laparoscopic colon resection has only been attempted in 19% of the hospitals.

To date, approximately 150 laparoscopic bowel resections have been performed in The Netherlands. In order to report on their first experiences, surgeons from 5 Dutch hospitals accumulated the results of their first 77 laparoscopic bowel procedures. These data from the Free University Hospital Amsterdam (M.A. Cuesta), St. Antonius Hospital Nieuwegein (A. Jansen), St. Clara Hospital (J.F. Lange), Alkmaar Medical Center (B. Bijnen), and University Hospital, Maastricht (P.M.N.Y.H. Go) will be reported in this paper. Special attention is focussed on local recurrences and port-site recurrences after resection for bowel cancer. The latter is considered a problem associated with laparoscopic resection.

Laparoscopic resection is a challenge for the surgeon. A promising instrument, the laparoscopic ultrasonic dissector is described as an aid for 'tissue selective' dissection. In laparoscopy, one lacks palpation, e.g. to detect liver metastasis. Laparoscopic ultrasonography can be an aid to replace surgical palpation. Both instruments will be described briefly.

National Survey

In the period July 1991 to December 1992 surgeons in 5 hospitals performed 77 laparoscopic bowel procedures. These include ileocecal resection, right hemicolectomy, sigmoid resection, anterior resection, restoration of bowel continuity after a Hartmann's procedure, and posterior rectopexy. In 38 patients resections were performed for large

Peter M.N.Y.H. Go, MD, PhD
Department of Surgery
St. Antonius Hospital
PO Box 2500
NL–3430 CM Nieuwegein (The Netherlands)

0253–4886/95/0125–0277
$ 8.00/0

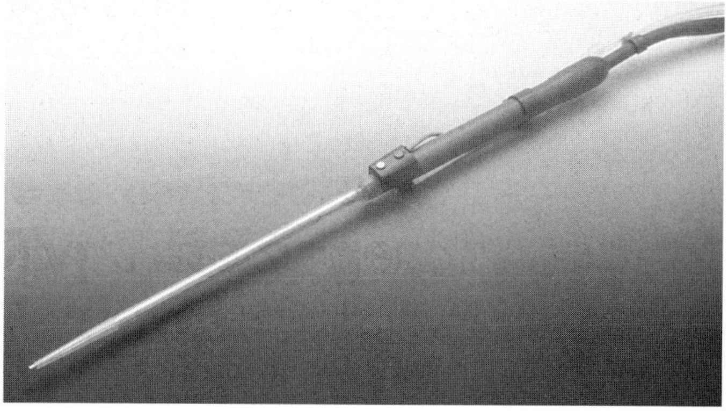

Fig. 1. Laparoscopic ultrasonic dissector in combination with electrosurgery: Laparoscopic CUSA® (Valleylab Inc., Boulder, Colo., USA).

Table 1. Data of laparoscopic bowel operations in The Netherlands collected from 5 institutions

Procedure type	n	Average age years	Average operation time, min	Postoperative hospital stay, days
Ileocecal resection	3	–	180	7
Right hemicolectomy	19	69	240	10
Sigmoid resection	36	64	210	8
Anterior resection	6	59	290	9
Reanastomosis after Hartmann's procedure	10	67	190	10
Posterior rectopexy	3	63	220	6

bowel cancer. The sex ratio was 1:1. The average follow-up at evaluation was 10 (3–17) months. The following items were evaluated: operation time, reasons for conversion to laparotomy, postoperative hospital stay, complications and costs of additional disposable laparoscopic instruments.

In table 1 the number of patients per procedure type, their average age, the operation time, and the postoperative hospital stay are given. The operation time is longer than for the conventional operation, but the average postoperative hospital stay is from the Dutch perspective relatively short. Conversion to laparotomy was necessary in 17% of the patients. The reasons were: severe adhesions (7), inadequate exposure (2), severe inflammation (2), and bowel lesion due to instrumentation (2). There was no mortality. Anastomotic leak occurred in 1 patient after reanastomosis after Hartmann's procedure. Another patient had an ileus immediately postoperatively due to 360° rotation of the bowel at the anastomotic site, which was found at laparotomy. Infectious complications consist of one intraabdominal abscess and one wound infection. Two patients had an anastomotic stenosis 3 months postoperatively. The use of disposable laparoscopic instruments add an average of USD 1,600 per procedure.

All 38 patients operated on for bowel cancer had free resection margins. On average 9.2 (SD 2.5) lymph nodes were found in the resected specimens. No local recurrences were noticed during the 10 months follow-up. In 2 institutions, 18 patients after laparoscopic bowel resections are followed for an average duration of 20 months. In this group 6 patients died of distant metastasis. The remaining 12 patients are still alive and have no signs of local recurrence. In two other centers 3 of 36 patients had subcutaneous metastasis. These recurrences occurred at the specimen removal site (2) and at a distant trocar site (1) [1]. Port-site metastasis seems to be a particular concern in laparoscopic bowel resection for cancer. Wexner and Cohen [2] found an incidence of 6.3% in a literature review. This percentage is higher than in conventional colectomies. A possible mechanism is direct implantation of viable tumor cells during extraction of the tissue specimen through a small incision [3]. Prudence is therefore called for laparoscopic bowel resection for cancer, which should be done along with a clinical trial. Furthermore, controlled randomized trials should be done to assess the place of laparoscopy in bowel resections [3].

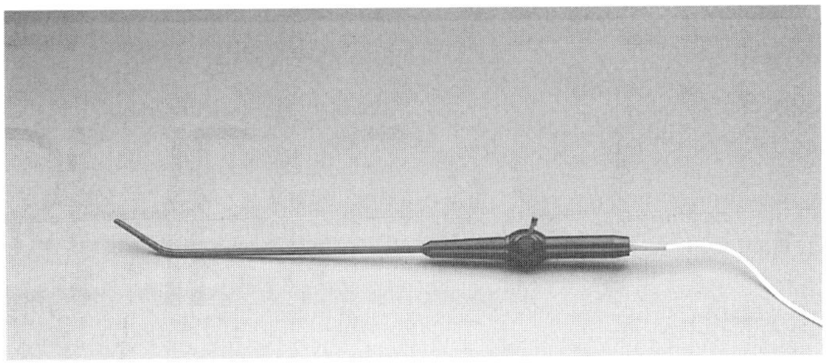

Fig. 2. Laparoscopic ultrasonography probe, linear array, 7.5 MHz, with a steerable tip (Pie Medical, Maastricht, The Netherlands).

Two Instruments for Laparoscopic Colon Operations

As mentioned before, laparoscopic colectomy is an advanced laparoscopic procedure that is time consuming. New technology can be an aid to facilitate the operation. The laparoscopic ultrasonic dissector is such a device (fig. 1). An acoustic vibrator is coupled to a titanium tip that oscillates at 23,000 cpm. The ultrasound waves create cavitation effect in tissues with high water contents such as parenchymatous and fatty tissue. Fibrous and collagenous tissue, such as blood vessels, are less affected. This results in tissue selectivity during dissection, where fatty tissue of the mesocolon is dissected and blood vessels are spared. The tip is irrigated with saline that increases the cavitation effect. Aspiration through the hollow tip allows removal of debris. The combination with electrosurgery adds coagulation properties to the device. The device is especially helpful for mesocolon dissection [4].

In laparoscopy, the surgeon lacks palpation of the intraabdominal organs. During bowel cancer resection the liver is palpated for the presence of liver metastasis. One way to replace the surgeon's palpation during the laparoscopic operation is ultrasonography. Figure 2 shows a laparoscopic probe that fits through a 10-mm port. It is a 7.5-Mhz linear array probe with a steerable tip. The tip is directly applied to the liver surface showing high-resolution images. The whole liver can then be scanned for metastasis. By combining the ultrasonic images with laparoscopic image using picture-in-picture facilities, an exact location of abnormalities can be determined. In addition, histology can be obtained by puncture biopsies under ultrasonic guidance. Calculation of sensitivity and specificity to detect liver metastases from colon carcinoma with laparoscopic ultrasonography need further evaluation.

Conclusion

In this paper, preliminary results are presented from laparoscopic bowel resections in The Netherlands. They are encouraging, although the occurrence of a relatively high percentage of port-site subcutaneous metastasis in cancer surgery is alarming. In The Netherlands, plans are being made to join an international randomized controlled trial to determine the place of laparoscopy in bowel resections for cancer.

References

1 Berends FJ, Kazemier G, Bonjer HJ, Lange JF: Subcutaneous metastasis after laparoscopic colectomy. Lancet 1994;344:58.

2 Wexner SD, Cohen SM: Port site metastasis after laparoscopic colorectal surgery for cure of malignancy. Br J Surg 1995;82:295–298.

3 Monson JRT, Hill ADK, Darzi A: Laparoscopic colon surgery. Br J Surg 1995;82:150–157.

4 Go PMNYH: Ultrasonic dissection and monopolar coagulation: A new device in laparoscopic treatment of gastrointestinal cancer; in Cuesta MA, Nagy AG (eds): Minimally Invasive Surgery in Gastrointestinal Cancer. Edinburgh, Churchill Livingstone, 1993, pp 26–31.

Dig Surg 1995;12:280–283

A. Fingerhut
B. Millat
P. Lointier
J.M. Hay

Association de Recherche en Chirurgie;
Association de Recherche Universitaire en Chirurgie,
Association de Recherche en Chirurgie de l'Ile de France,
Association de Recherche en Chirurgie Viscérale du Languedoc, France

Is Laparoscopic Colonic Resection for Carcinoma Feasible and Safe?

A French Collective Experience

Key Words
Carcinoma · Colonic resection · Laparoscopy

In contrary to other laparoscopic procedures, colonic resection, accomplished more and more frequently under videolaparoscopic control [1], has given rise to increasing controversy and concern. The advantages found for laparoscopic cholecystectomy such as shorter hospital stay, less postoperative pain and ileus [2], or quicker return to normal activity [1, 3, 4] have not been shown in laparoscopic colonic resection. We present herein a prospective experience of 163 unselected laparoscopic colonic resections for carcinoma, performed by surgeons in the French Associations for Research in Surgery and analyze the results as regards the hypothetical advantages over traditional colonic resections.

Patients and Methods

During an 18-month period (October 1991 to March 1994), 163 patients (mean age = 68.5 ± 11.4; range: 14–94 years), 94 females and 69 males, were potential candidates for laparoscopic colonic resection for carcinoma (n = 94; 57.7%), 62 polyps or villous tumors (38%), completion colectomy for appendicular carcinoid in 3, appendicular mucocele in 1, and 3 cases of familial polyposis.

Results

Overall, there were 53 conversions (33%). The reasons were: (1) difficulties or accidents during dissection (for instance wounding of the iliac artery in one case): 27 cases, 17% (including 5 cases of exceedingly voluminous tumor); (2) impossibility of creating or maintaining carboperitoneum in 2 cases; (3) difficulty to perform the anastomosis in 5 cases (3%). The operation was discontinued in 5 cases because the surgeon had gone over the time limit he had fixed for himself to perform the operation. In 9 cases, the conversion was motivated for carcinological reasons including impossibility of performing adequate lymph node dissection in 2 cases, difficulties in dissection because of tumor extension in 3, impossibility of locating the tumor or the endoscopic resection site in 2 cases each, while the reason for conversion was not given in 1 case.

There was a total of 110 completed laparoscopic procedures. The mean delay of operation (laparoscopic only) was 206 ± 80 min (range 60–600). The mean time to return of intestinal activity was 2.9 days (range 10 h to 8 days). Postoperative analgesics were necessary for a mean of 2.8 days (range 0–10). There were 13 (8%) anastomotic fistulas,

Abe Fingerhut, MD
Centre Hospitalier Intercommunal
10, rue du Champ-Gaillard
F–78303 Poissy (France)

0253–4886/95/0125–0280
$ 8.00/0

two radiological only. Seven patients died (five fistulas). The mean hospital stay was 13.8 (6–76) days. Of 82 available pathology reports, the mean length of distal tumor clearance was 6.3 ± 5 cm (range 0–24). In 56% of cases, the distal margin was 5 cm or less. The mean number of lymph nodes removed per specimen was 6.1 (0–37). In six specimens (13%), no lymph nodes were found at all.

There were 3 cases of early recurrence (less than 3 months) and 2 postoperative obstructions due to missed (second) tumors. Last, there were 3 cases of tumor seeding at trocar sites (two Dukes C and one Dukes B) (3% of cancers stage B, C, and D).

Discussion

In spite of the scarcity of true comparative trials on the subject, laparoscopic surgery has been shown to reduce operative insult and to ameliorate the quality of recovery, notably after cholecystectomy [3, 5]. Although some authors have stated that the same may be expected after colonic surgery [6, 7], this type of resection is technically more demanding. New and preoccupying problems have arisen including tissue handling [4] and increased morbidity, proper identification of tumor and extension [2], difficulty of anastomosis and removal of resected tissues from the abdomen [4], dissemination of disease on the peritoneum and at trocar sites [8–12], as well as the now classical but probably more difficult learning curve [13].

Imperfect technique in laparoscopic surgery is recognized to increase the morbidity rate [14] as well as, in carcinoma, the recurrence rate [15, 16]. Adequate tissue resection is essential in colonic resection for malignancy [17] and must not be compromised by minimal invasive surgery at all costs [4, 16, 18]. Several reports have emphasized equivalent mesenteric, nodal, and longitudinal resection of malignant colorectal disease [4, 6, 7, 18]. However, there have been little if any reports on the circumferential margins which, if positive, are associated with a local recurrence rate as high as 87% in open surgery [16]. It is to be hoped that modern imaging such as magnetic resonance, transluminal ultrasound and immunoscintigraphy will enable the surgeon to better detect locally invasive tumors and to determine the proper indications for laparoscopic or conventional surgery [18].

Carcinoma seeding at the sites of trocar insertion after laparoscopy has been reported with increasing frequency after resection for colonic carcinoma. The risk in open surgery has been estimated to be 0.7% (11 patients with recurrence associated with the laparotomy incision or drainage site in 1,603 patients) [19], but only sporadic cases have been observed in colonic resection. As recurrence can occur in sites which have not been used for the extraction of the specimen, this leads one to speculate that direct dissemination is not the cause and that simply enveloping the specimen in a plastic bag for extraction is not sufficient to avoid this. It is well known that manipulation of tumor can cause viable malignant cells to exfoliate [20, 21] and to implant and then grow in healing colonic anastomosis. Also, it is known since 1914 that tumor cell growth is enhanced by tissue injury and that, through the circulation, tumor cells can seed in injured tissues [22] or the laparotomy wound [23]. Skipper et al. [12] have determined experimentally that enhanced proliferation is 1,000-fold in the healing tissues. Moreover, their dispersion into the port sites may in some way be facilitated by the carboperitoneum [18].

The number of lymph nodes cleared with specimens is thought to be of prognostic importance. Retrieval of lymph nodes in the mesentery or at the origin of the inferior mesenteric vein in left colonic carcinoma [24], while not influencing outcome, can help determine the stage of disease before deciding whether further adjuvant therapy is necessary or not. Laparoscopically, Philips et al. [7] reported an average yield of 14 (range 8–22) in their 24 cases, higher than the amounts published by Vara Thorbeck et al. [2] (mean = 8.5; range 7–12) and our series, but much lower than the 34 (range 0–88) found per specimen by Herrera et al. [25] in open surgery. The number of lymph node metastases found obviously increases with the number of lymph nodes examined [25, 26] and is known to differ according to patient anatomy, individual surgical expertise and technique and above all with the interest generated by pathologists to search for them [25].

Missed tumors have not been reported often. One of 18 patients in the series of Vara-Thorbeck et al. [2] had to undergo a standard resection of a Dukes' B2 tumor 10 cm from the anastomosis 9 months after the initial colonic resection. McDermott et al. [27] reported another case of unrecognized synchronous cancer revealed by obstruction 2 weeks after initial left colectomy. Synchronous cancer is reported in up to 5% of the cases [28]. Colonoscopy has a false-negative rate of 3–8% [28, 29]. As manual palpation is difficult or impossible in laparoscopic surgery (for the colonic tumor as well as for hepatic metastases), this leads us to conclude that complete workup is necessary before engaging on laparoscopic resection. In the absence of such workup or when the expected tumor site is not confirmed, preoperative tattooing and/or intraoperative colonoscopy should be entertained.

Our fistula rate (9.5%) may seem surprising, but anastomotic failure rates as high as 18% have been reported in laparoscopic surgery [7]. Infection increases the mortality, perioperative and late morbidity, as well as promotes recurrence [30]. In multivariate analysis, our research group [unpubl. data] showed that intraoperative contamination was a predictive factor of fistula. Anastomoses performed under videolaparoscopy are usually closed; the preparation was the same, but it is more difficult to clamp the intestines or protect the operative field. The lower rates reported in the literature often concern surgical 'centers of excellence', and which, as such, probably recruit and operate on selected patients. This multicenter report is most likely closer to reality as colonic surgery in France (as in most other countries) is performed by qualified surgeons from university and general hospitals as well as private clinics and not only in specialized centers.

It has been stated that return of postoperative bowel function and length of hospital stay are shorter in patients undergoing laparoscopic colonic resection as compared with conventional surgery [7]. This was not confirmed by the Cleveland Clinic group [1] or Milsom et al. [31], nor our study. More recently, a prospective randomized trial from the Cleveland Clinic has shown that early oral intake (less than 24 h after surgery) was well tolerated after laparotomy and that early feeding after surgery was not limited to laparoscopy [32]. Moreover, the possibility of earlier discharge is theoretical at most and may well be related to sociocultural and financial factors.

Conclusions

Laparoscopic colonic resections and anastomoses have been shown to be feasible. In this report, however, we found that morbidity was increased, abdominal and intestinal exploration were difficult and carcinologic rules were not always respected in the population of patients studied. As others [8], we cannot recommend laparoscopic surgery for colonic carcinoma at present. Although some institutions are continuing to perform colonic surgery for carcinoma, others have restricted their indications to benign disease and/or premalignant (adenoma) or malignant lesions requiring minimal or limited resections [7], or to patients with incurable disease or those with contraindications to standard surgery [2]. Improvement of laparoscopic skills in the general surgical community, of instrumentation as well as techniques of localization, are certainly necessary. Further investigation of the possible enhancement of carcinologic seeding by laparoscopic techniques is also needed. As noncontrolled trials performed to date do not seem to show any difference in length of hospital stay or a decrease of postoperative pain as compared with standard techniques, as morbidity seems high, and carcinological rules difficult to adhere to because of technical constraints, there is a definite need for controlled trials to determine if laparoscopic colonic resection should be continued in the cancer setting and if they are of any real benefit to the patient.

References

1 Wexner SD, Cohen SM, Johansen OB, Nogguera JJ, Jagelman DG: Laparoscopic colorectal surgery: A prospective assessment and current perspective. Br J Surg 1993;80:1602–1605.

2 Vara-Thorbeck C, Garcia-Caballero M, Salvi M, Gutstein D, Toscano R, Gomez A, Vara-Thorbeck R: Indications and advantages of laparoscopy-assisted colon resection for carcinoma in elderly patients. Surg Lapar Endosc 1994;4:110–118.

3 Barkun JS, Barkun AN, Sampalis JS, Fried G, Taylor B, Wexler MJ, Goresky CA, Meakins J: Randomized controlled trial of laparoscopic versus mini-cholecystectomy. Lancet 1992;340:1116–1119.

4 Tate JJT, Kwok S, Dawson JW, Lau WY, Li AKC: Prospective comparison of laparoscopic and conventional anterior resection. Br J Surg 1993;80:1396–1398.

5 Reddick EJ, Olsend DO: Laparoscopic laser cholecystectomy: A comparison with minilaparotomy cholecystectomy. Surg Endosc 1989;3:131–133.

6 Monson JRT, Darzi A, Carey PDD, Guillou PJ: Prospective evaluation of laparoscopic-assisted colectomy in an unselected group of patients; Lancet 1992;340:831–833.

7 Phillips EH, Franklin M, Cartoll BJ, Fallas MJ, Ramos R, Rosenthal D: Laparoscopic colectomy. Ann Surg 1992;216:703–707.

8 Alexander RJT, Jacques BC, Mitchell KG: Laparoscopically assisted colectomy and wound recurrence. Lancet 1993;341:249–250.

9 Fusco MA, Paluzzi MW: Abdominal wall recurrence after laparoscopic assisted colectomy for adenocarcinoma of the colon. Dis Colon Rectum 1993;36:858–861.

10 Nduka CC, Monson JRT, Menzies-Gow N, Darzi A: Abdominal wall metastases following laparoscopy. Br J Surg 1994;81:648–652.

11 O'Rourke N, Price PM, Kelly S, Sikora K: Tumour inoculation during laparoscopy (letter). Lancet 1993;342:368.

12 Skipper D, Jeffrey MJ, Cooper AJ, Alexander P, Taylor I: Enhanced growth of tumour cells in healing colonic anastomoses and laparotomy wounds. Int J Colorectal Dis 1989;4:172–177.

13 Pappas TN: Laparoscopic colectomy – the innovation continues. Ann Surg 1992;216:701–702.

14 Chamberlain G, Brown J: Report of the Working Party of the Confidential Enquiry into Gynaecological Laparoscopy. London, Royal College of Obstetricians & Gynaecologists, 1978.

15 Fielding LP, Stewart-Brown S, Dudly HAF: Surgeon-related variables and the clinical trial. Lancet 1986;ii:778–779.

16 Quirke P, Durdey P, Dixon MF, Williams NS: Local recurrence of rectal adenocarcinoma due to inadequate surgical resection. Lancet 1986;ii:996–999.

17 Michiels C, Boutron MC, Chatelain N, Quinpourt V, Roy P, Faivre J: Facteurs pronostiques des adénocarcinomes colorectaux de stade B de Dukes: Etude d'une série de population. Gastroentérol Clin Biol 1994;18:456–461.
18 Guillou PJ: Laparoscopic surgery for diseases of the colon and rectum quo vadis? Surg Endosc 1994;8:669–671.
19 Hughes ES, McDermott FT, Polgase AI, Johnson WR: Tumor recurrence in the abdominal wall scar tissue after large bowel cancer bowel surgery. Dis Colon Rectum 1982;26:571–572.
20 Fermor B, Umpleby HC, Lever JV, Symes MO, Williamson RC: Proliferative and metastatic potential of exfoliated colorectal carcinoma cells. Br J Surg 1984;71:659–663.
21 Umpleby HC, Fermor B, Symes MO, Williamson RCN: Viability of exfoliated colorectal carcinoma cells. Br J Surg 1984;71: 659–663.
22 Alexander JW, Altemeier WA: Susceptibility of injured tissues to haematogenous metastases; an experimental study. Ann Surg 1964; 85:933–944.
23 Murphy P, Alexander P, Senior PV, Fleming J, Kirkham N, Taylor I: Mechanisms of organ selective tumour growth by bloodborne cancer cells. Br J Cancer 1988;57:19–31.
24 Saclarides TJ, Ko ST, Airan M, Dillon C, Franklin J: Laparoscopic removal of a large colonic lipoma. Dis Colon Rectum 1991;34: 1027–1029.
25 Herrera L, Villarreal JR: Incidence of metastases from rectal adenocarcinoma in small lymph nodes detected by a clearing technique. Dis Colon Rectum 1992;35:783–788.
26 Cawthorn SJ, Gibbs NM, Marks CG: Clearance technique for the detection of lymph nodes in colorectal cancer. Br J Surg 1986;73: 58–60.
27 McDermott JP, Devereaux DA, Caushaj PF: Pitfall of laparoscopic colectomy: An unrecognized synchronous cancer. Dis Colon Rectum 1994;37:602–603.
28 Byrd RL, Boggs HW, Stragle GW, Cole PA: Reliability of colonoscopy. Dis Colon Rectum 1989;32:1023–1025.
29 Abrams JS: A hard look at colonoscopy. Am J Surg 1977;133:111.
30 Sauven P, Playforth MJ, Evans M, Pollock AV: Early infective complications and late recurrent cancer in stapled colonic anastomoses. Dis Colon Rectum 1989;32:33–35.
31 Milsom JW, Iavery IC, Church JM, Stolfi VM, Fazio VW: Use of laparoscopic techniques in colorectal surgery: Preliminary study. Dis Colon Rectum 1994;37:215–218.
32 Binderow SR, Cohen SM, Wexner SD: Must early postoperative oral intake be limited to laparoscopy? Dis Colon Rectum 1994;37: 584–589.

Dig Surg 1995;12:284–287

Morris E. Franklin Jr.
San Antonio, Tex., USA

Laparoscopic Management of Colorectal Disease

The United States Experience

Key Words
Colorectal disease · Laparoscopic management · Indications · Technique · Training

I unfortunately do not have information to relay to you the entire United States experience in laparoscopic colon surgery; however, I would like to give you the experience of two relatively large centers that perform a great number of colon and rectal surgeries laparoscopically.

Diagnostic laparoscopy began in 1910 with initial gynecological procedures being performed in the 1930s. Definitive gynecological procedures of a therapeutic nature were performed in the 1960s but these were primarily tubal ligations. Therapeutic procedures, particularly oophorectomy, lysis of adhesions, and care of patients with ectopic pregnancies began in earnest in the 1980s. Initial general surgery laparoscopic procedures began in the mid-1980s, but were again primarily of a diagnostic nature although Curt Simms did report a large series of appendectomies for primarily non inflammatory disease during this period of time. The first laparoscopic cholecystectomy was performed by Mouel in 1987, and the first laparoscopic cholecystectomy was performed in the United States in 1988 by McKernan and then very shortly thereafter by Reddick. The first laparoscopic colon resection procedures were performed in 1980 primarily as laparoscopic mobilization by Jacobs and Placencia and totally intracorporeal laparoscopic colon resection for carcinoma was in 1990 by Franklin. The demonstrated advantages of laparoscopic surgery include less pain, shortened hospitalization, quicker recovery, quicker return to normal function, a virtual lack of wound problems, quicker institution of adjuvant therapy as well as a thorough visual evaluation of the abdominal cavity. The perceived disadvantages of laparoscopic surgery include specialized equipment, advanced training, and increased cost of OR as opposed to hospitalization versus recovery. When these are considered in toto laparoscopic surgery is perhaps less expensive. A question has arisen as to whether laparoscopic procedures are applicable to all disease processes. Another perceived disadvantage of laparoscopic surgery is loss of palpatory sense and one of the primary complaints about laparoscopic surgery is that the anatomy appears different from a laparoscopic viewpoint compared to open. In reality, the anatomy is not different; however, it does have a different appearance laparoscopically.

The indications for laparoscopic colorectal surgery include diagnostic procedures used to differentiate appendicitis from diverticulitis or perforated viscous. Staging of carcinoma has been utilized to some extent laparoscopically but has not been widely accepted. Inflammatory diseases of the bowel including diverticulitis, Crohn's disease, and ulcerative colitis have all been approached successfully laparoscopically with varying degrees of success. Other indications for laparoscopic colorectal surgery include the care of polyps (adenomatous, villous adenoma, and familia polyposis) utilizing segmental resections as well as polyp-

Morris E. Franklin, Jr., MD, FACS
4242 E. South Cross #4
San Antonio, TX 78222 (USA)

0253–4886/95/0125–0284
$ 8.00/0

ectomy. Additional indications include bleeding from a diverticular source, arteriovenous malformations, and, on rare occasions, ischemia. An ideal indication for laparoscopic colorectal surgery in particular reported by Wexner and Stitz in Australia has been in the care of patients with dysmotility problems many times with subtotal colectomy with or without an anastomosis. Other indications for laparoscopic colorectal surgery include volvulus and reestablishing continuity where an ostomy has been performed. The question of laparoscopic approach to cancer has been a subject of tremendous debate and the debate continues. Several centers worldwide have established definite criteria and have shown outstanding results in the care of cancer patients of all stages with a laparoscopic approach.

The contraindications for laparoscopic colorectal surgery are very often surgeon dependent. However, certain general rules apply in consideration of any patient for a laparoscopic colorectal procedure. The accepted contraindications for laparoscopic colorectal surgery include inability to tolerate general anesthesia, bleeding dyscrasias, and advanced liver disease with ascites. This latter category is certainly a relative contraindication as we have operated on many patients with advanced liver disease with ascites and have successfully taken them through their operations. Severe cardiac pulmonary disease has been sighted on a recurrent basis as a reason for avoiding laparoscopic surgery. We have found, however, as time goes on that these are the kind of patients who benefit the most from laparoscopic and minimally invasive approaches, despite whatever disease process might be present.

Other relative contraindications for laparoscopic colorectal procedures include multiple operations with known severe adhesions. A large tumor with extensive involvement, including a frozen pelvis or right upper quadrant where debulking procedures are considered advantageous is best approached with an open surgical procedure. Along the same vein, adjacent organ spread of carcinoma is an additional relative contraindication depending on the organ involved and the experience and expertise of the surgeon. We have successfully excised numerous tumors which have invaded the bladder and included in the procedure a partial cystectomy with a successful primary closure of the bladder. The presence of a large abdominal aortic aneurysm should always alert the would be laparoscopic surgeon to the possibility of a difficult dissection, particularly if the aneurysm is in the region of the origin of the inferior mesenteric artery and/or the bifurcation of the aorta. In this instance, visualization of all structures may be nearly impossible and this type of patient should be considered for an open procedure.

The types of procedures which we have performed laparoscopically include laparoscopic polypectomy with a colotomy and excision of the polyp although we have for the most part abandoned this procedure. A primary use of laparoscopy is that of a laparoscopic monitored colonoscopic polypectomy where with a large sessile polyp an unprotected colonoscopic excision is considered hazardous. In this instance a laparoscopy is performed, the involved segment of the colon is mobilized and isolated, the colonoscope is brought into the colon and under direct vision a colonoscopic polypectomy is performed with direct visualization of the wall of the colon via the laparoscope. This has resulted in a remarkable improvement in the ability to perform these procedures colonoscopically. Construction of ostomies in the case of perforation with peritonitis and/or obstruction is readily performed laparoscopically. Ostomies can also be closed with relative ease once the surgeon becomes skilled in these procedures. Segmental resection of any portion of the colon can readily be accomplished with a laparoscopically assisted or a totally intracorporeal technique. Total colectomies as well as APRs are approached laparoscopically but are quite dependent on the skills of the operating surgeon and of the specific disease process.

The equipment needed for laparoscopic colon surgery include the standard vidioscopic equipment utilized for advanced laparoscopic procedures of any kind. However, a multiple positional table is virtually a mandatory item of equipment for successful laparoscopic colon surgery. The table must be able to be placed in severe Trendelenburg, reverse Trendelenburg with a left and right tilt, and have ability for adequate anal access on all cases. An adequate laparoscope and video camera, preferably of a 3-chip variety, are also very helpful in successful completion of these types of procedures. A colonoscope should be readily available with a monitor that can be viewed both by the operating surgeon as well as the colonoscopist. A variety of special laparoscopic hand-held instruments, including laparoscopic Babcocks, 10-mm scissors, laparoscopic allyces, and laparoscopic Glassman clamps are also of extreme help. Electrocoagulation capabilities must be present, however the presence of a laser is not necessarily recommended for laparoscopic procedures. An argon beam coagulator can be of extreme help particularly with low anterior resections where troublesome bleeding from presacral vessels presents a problem. Included also in the list of equipment should be a sterile specimen bag which can be used to encompass an infected specimen and/or a carcinomatous specimen which might shed tumor cells and/or bacteria into extraction sites or in the case of transanal extraction, along the anal canal. Also included in necessary laparoscopic equipment for colon resection is that of endoscopic stapling, cutting, suturing, and anastomotic equipment including on occasion special bulldog Glassman clamps for occluding the bowel and/or controlling blood vessels.

The technique for laparoscopic colon and rectal procedures of course depends on the segment of the colon upon which an operation is to be performed. There are some general rules which apply to all patients, however, that is the patient should be supine, there should be anal access, and the patient should be secured to the table for positional changes. Nasogastric tube, Foley catheter, and sequential compression devices should be in place. We strongly advocate patient monitoring including CO_2, temperature and arterial blood gas determinations as needed. All techniques are begun with insufflation. This can be done with a Veress needle or with Hesson-type techniques. A laparoscopy is then performed, the diseased segment is identified, and is mobilized extensively. The blood supply to the given segment of colon should be thoroughly identified and a determination should be made if control of the vascular structure is to be performed intracorporeally or extracorporeally. We recommend intracorporeal control of all blood vessels in the case of carcinoma and have found this to be advantageous in benign disease processes as well. Adjacent structures in and near the given segment of colon should be identified very thoroughly. We feel it is mandatory to identify both left and right ureters in all low anterior and sigmoid resections. Nonidentification of the ureters should immediately evoke opening of the patient. The bladder and major blood vessels in the area should also be identified and a thorough knowledge of the anatomy in the area is mandatory for successful laparoscopic colon surgery. In the case of the right colon, the location of the duodenum should be utmost in the surgeon's mind and definite identification of the duodenum should be made early in the process. After the segment of colon has been very thoroughly mobilized, a resection is then carried out either with a stapling and cutting technique, with ligation or even on occasion opening of the colon with immediate closure of the proximal and distal ends of the resected portion of the colon. The specimen can also be resected from the outside of the abdomen by thoroughly mobilizing the diseased segment of the colon and bringing it through a small incision and completing the resection outside of the body. The specimen can be removed by a number of routes. Basically, these amount to either removal through a natural orifice such as a transanal or transvaginal site or through an accessory incision. We feel strongly that all specimens, particularly those of an infectious or inflammatory nature or those with carcinoma, should be placed in a specimen bag for safe removal.

Laparoscopic anastomosis can be performed by a number of techniques. The simplest anastomosis is that of an extracorporeal anastomosis where the proximal and distal ends of a given segment of bowel are brought to the surface and a hand-sewn or stapled anastomosis is completed completely extracorporeally. This is probably the most popular form of anastomosis for right hemicolectomy. A laparoscopically assisted anastomosis which is partly intracorporeal, is the next most popular procedure and is most useful in low anterior and sigmoid resections where the proximal end of the colon is brought out to the abdominal wall and an anvil inserted. The anvil is replaced in the abdominal cavity, the wound closed, and the abdomen is then reinsufflated. The distal end of the colon has been previously stapled and the head of the stapler is brought into the rectum and the two portions of the stapler are reconnected. This is a virtually mandatory procedure for patients undergoing low anterior and low sigmoid resections where each end of the colon can not be brought to the surface. The most difficult but perhaps the most efficacious anastomosis is that of a totally intracorporeal anastomosis where additional incisions are not made for mere placement of the anvil. In the instance of sigmoid resections, the anvil is brought through the rectum, placed into the proximal bowel, the proximal bowel is then closed with staples or endoloops, the excess tissue is trimmed and the anvil is then readied for completion of the stapling procedure as outlined in the laparoscopically assisted procedures. For right colon resections a quadruple stapled anastomosis can readily be fashioned and functions quite well as a totally intracorporeal anastomosis. We feel very strongly that all anastomoses should be tested and that intraoperative colonoscopy should be performed both to test the anastomosis, to check for leaks, and to be assured that there is no bleeding from the anastomotic staple line.

The results of laparoscopic colon surgery are of course dependent upon the operator and most particularly upon his experience. The results presented herein will be of the two largest series in the United States: that of Jacobs and Placensia from Miami, and my results from San Antonio, Tex. In the Miami experience, Moises Jacobs and Gus Pacensia have now performed more than 235 colon procedures, 75 have been for diverticular disease, 30 for benign polyps, and 130 for carcinoma. Their postoperative hospital stay if the patient is under 50 years of age has averaged 3.7 days. If patients are over 50 years of age it is 5.7 days. Their wound complication rate has run 2%, anastomotic complication rate has also been 2%. They have had a 15% conversion to open. Plasencia and Jacobs have at the time of this writing had no incidence of trocar site implications in their primarily operated patients who are less than stage IV carcinoma. All operations have been performed by Jacobs and Plasencia who have repeatedly exhibited their skill as outstanding laparoscopic surgeons.

Another large series is that of the Texas Endosurgery Institute in San Antonio, Tex., with the primary surgeon being myself. Here we have performed 215 resections including 53 for diverticular disease, 3 for benign polyps, 145 for carcinoma of all stages, 4 for bleeding, and 10 total colectomies. We also have almost 100 non-resectional procedures including 28 monitored colonoscopic polypectomies, 22 polypectomies, 10 ostomies constructed and 30+ ostomy closures. The hospital days for the TEI patients if they are less than 50 years of age is 3.5 days; if they are over 50 years old 7.25 days. We have had 2 of 315 patients with wound complications, 6 of 215 with anastomotic complications, and have converted 12 of 315 to open for a 3.8% rate. To this date, we have had at the Texas Endosurgery Institute, 4 deaths, all related to basic cardiovascular disease which many of our patients have had. We have also had 1 instance of pneumonia resulting in death at 21 days postoperation. We have had several urinary tract infections related to indwelling catheters, and have had delayed ileus resulting in delay of postoperative feedings for up to 5 days in 4 patients. We have reoperated on 4 patients, 2 for bleeding, 1 for suspected abscess where none was found, and 1 for a suspected anastomotic leak where ileostomy was performed. There have been in our series, particularly with carcinoma patients, no trocar implants in primarily resected patients of all stages. We have a very careful follow-up on all of our patients who have undergone totally intracorporeal resection for carcinoma and have found that the complication rate, life span and incidence of recurrent carcinoma have all been the same or better than a well-documented group of patients who have had open surgery by a well-known colorectal group in San Antonio. The primary difference in these two groups is that (1) there has been a lack of wound complications in the laparoscopic group; (2) the patients were able to go home much quicker, and (3) they are able to return to normal activities much sooner than those patients undergoing open colon resection. The number of lymph nodes and the margins of resection have been exactly the same or perhaps greater in the laparoscopic group.

Trocar implantations have been a worldwide problem and a concern of all laparoscopic as well as open colon surgeons. It appears that trocar implantations are related to experience as well as to the disease process. I am aware of 44 trocar implantations worldwide. Most of these have been either at an extraction site or in the first 10 patients who had been operated on by a given colorectal surgeon. I have accumulated 1,100 cases of colon cancer that have been operated upon by laparoscopic means in the hands of experienced surgeons and to date there have been no trocar implantations in this group.

In conclusion, laparoscopy has opened a new arena for treatment for most colon and rectal diseases, however multiple issues are present in this new and exciting field. These include technique, training, and the approach to carcinoma. There is no doubt that an extremely high level of skill is needed to successfully complete these procedures and many excellent open surgeons will never to be able to successfully perform this surgery. The exact role of laparoscopy in the treatment of carcinoma is yet to be determined although the preliminary results from several large centers have indeed been encouraging.

References

1 Jacobs M, Verdeja GD, Goldstein DS: Minimally invasive colon resection. Surg Laparosc Endosc 1992;2:144–150.

2 Franklin ME, Rosenthal D, Ramos R: Laparoscopic colectomy: Utopia or reality? Gastrointest Clin North Am 1993;3:353–365.

3 Phillips EH, Franklin ME, Carroll BJ: Laparoscopic colectomy. Ann Surg 1991;216:703–707.

4 Franklin ME: Laparoscopic colon and small bowel surgery: Current techniques in Laparoscopy; in Brooks DC (ed): Current Medicine 1994.

5 Franklin ME, Rosenthal D, Norem R: Prospective Evaluation of Laparoscopic Colonic Resection Versus Open Colon Resection for Adenocarcinoma: A Multicenter Study. Surgical Endoscopy. New York, Springer, accepted.

Dig Surg 1995;12:288–292

F. Köckerling
C. Schneider
M.A. Reymond
Ch. Wittekind
Laparoscopic Colorectal Surgery Study Group

Surgical University Clinic,
Erlangen, Germany

Laparoscopic Colorectal Surgery: Indications and Concept of a Multicenter Study

Key Words
Laparoscopic colorectal surgery · Multicenter study

Introduction

Numerous problems are involved in the introduction of laparoscopic surgery into clinical practice (table 1). So far the published papers reported about the practicability, complication rates, lethality, short-term results and costs of laparoscopic colorectal surgery [1–7]. The introduction of laparoscopic operative techniques in colorectal cancer is thus discussed in a very controversial manner. On the one hand, the efficiency of laparoscopic colorectal surgery in carcinoma removal has not yet been established by long-term results, but on the other hand there are reports of metastases at the trocar placement area and at the port site [8–11]. For these reasons, the general use of laparoscopic surgical techniques for colorectal cancer cannot be recommended. Firstly, the values of these new operative techniques must be proven by the appropriate studies. Included in these special studies should be a pathological examination of the dissected tumor regarding its oncologic quality using an extended examination program as for example that used by the Study Group of the German Tumor Centers [12] (table 2).

Diagnostic and Palliative Laparoscopic Operations for Colorectal Cancer

There are no oncological principles against using explorative laparoscopy to exclude or confirm peritoneal or liver metastases (table 3). Nonresective procedures such as by-

Table 1. Laparoscopic colorectal surgery: problems

Extended lymph node dissection with high ligation of the inferior mesenteric artery, middle colic artery, right colic artery or iliocolic artery
Laparoscopic creation of a safe anastomosis
Specimen retrieval

Table 2. Prerequisites for curative laparoscopic oncological operations [12]

Histopathological examination of the tumor resection specimen for quality from an oncological standpoint must be guaranteed (extended examination program of the German Tumor Centers Study Group)
Recording and storage of long-term follow-up data by means of tumor follow-up in tumor centers or with a tumor registry must take place
⇒
As a rule, these prerequisites can only be fulfilled by special clinical studies

Table 3. Laparoscopic procedures for colorectal carcinoma which can be performed without observance of oncological principles

Explorative laparoscopy to exclude or confirm peritoneal or liver metastases
Nonresective procedures such as bypass operations or creation of a transverse colon stoma, a sigmoid colon stoma or a loop ileostomy
Palliative resections

Prof. Dr. med. F. Köckerling
Chirurgische Universitätsklinik
Postfach 35 60
D–91023 Erlangen (Germany)

0253–4886/95/0125–0288
$ 8.00/0

pass operations for advanced carcinoma of the left colon flexure with diffuse liver metastasis or creation of a transverse colon stoma, a sigmoid colon stoma or a loop ileostomy in advanced, metastasized colorectal cancer can also be performed laparoscopically [13–16]. Other indications for laparoscopy could be palliative colorectal resections or extirpation of the rectum in diffuse lung or liver metastasis. A very good argument for palliative treatment is that the patient's recovery is quicker and the length of hospitalization shorter. In cases of clearly poor prognosis of the cancer, palliative operative technique should be given preference over open surgery.

Table 4. Observance of oncological principles is technically unfeasible for the following laparoscopic colorectal resections

Anterior and deep anterior rectum resections
Distal transection of the rectum with an adequate margin of clearance from the tumor is too difficult
Tumor must be manipulated during dissection in the lesser pelvis
Right hemicolectomy
Identification of the ileocolic and right colic arteries on the trunk is difficult
Transection of the greater omentum and dissection in the area of the head of pancreas/duodenum is difficult
Extended colon resections

Technically Unfeasible Laparoscopic Colorectal Resections Under the Observance of Oncological Principles

A few operators who are very well experienced in laparoscopy have reported on the feasibility and excellent quality of deep anterior rectal resections and right-sided hemicolectomies for removal of carcinomas [17–22].

Taking experimental and clinical experiences of laparoscopic colorectal surgery into account, the operations have, depending on the anatomical site, proven to be rather difficult. Thus, dissection in a given anatomical layer is very possible, and with technical aids even reconstructive measures are successful in easily accessible anatomical regions; but there are technical and anatomical boundaries that can only be overcome by making concessions either for the oncological radicality or the safety of the operating procedure. For these reasons, we do not see any indication for carrying out laparoscopic anterior and deep anterior rectal resections in a multicenter study. Clean dissection of the mesorectum at the level of the removal line and distal resection of the rectum at a safe enough distance from the tumor is extremely difficult (table 4). In contrast to extirpation of the rectum, because the site of tumor dissection is deep in the pelvis, in cases of anterior and deep anterior rectal resection the tumor dissection has to be manipulated in the pelvis itself. Ligation of the inferior mesenteric artery at the trunk can be performed laparoscopically without any problem but necessitates extreme mobilization of the descending colon, the left colon flexure and the left-sided part of the transverse colon with resection of the transverse mesocolon from the underside of the pancreas and ligation of the inferior mesenteric vein at the lower border of the pancreas. Even these operative steps are technically very time-consuming and difficult laparoscopic maneuvers. Right-sided hemicolectomy or extended colon resections of flexure carcinomas are in our opinion also too complicated for the laparoscopic procedure and hold oncological risks. Firstly, finding the ileocolic artery and left colonic artery or middle colonic artery at the trunk is much more difficult and time-consuming carrying at the same time a higher risk of bleeding than the corresponding representation of the inferior mesenteric artery. Absence of the greater omentum from the large gastric curvature, opening of the omental bursa, resection of the transverse mesocolon, and the right colonic flexure from the duodenum and head of the pancreas are also in our opinion far too time-consuming. The relatively large right-sided colon carcinomas found frequently must be removed using minilaparatomy respective in size to the tumor.

Technically Feasible Laparoscopic Colorectal Resections of Carcinomas under the Observance of Oncological Principles

The technical and instrumental principles for carrying out good technically feasible laparoscopic colorectal resections under the observance of oncological principles are in our opinion indicated for small sigmoid carcinomas and for deeply situated rectal carcinomas that may only be reached by rectal extirpation for curative therapy [13, 17–25]. Transsection of the inferior mesenteric artery at the trunk is made possible by the preparatory representation and exteriorization of the arteries with a linear stapling device or PDS clips. Slight mobilization of the left colonic flexure for sigmoid resection is feasible. Retrieval in a specimen bag of a sigmoid resection of a small carcinoma is oncologically acceptable. A safe intracorporeal anastomosis can be achieved using conventional anastomosis techniques with purse string and circular stapler (table 5). In the course of the clinical studies as well as the examination of the indica-

Table 5. Observance of oncological principles is technically feasible in the following laparoscopic colorectal resections

Sigmoid resection	
	Transection of the inferior mesenteric artery at the trunk
	Mobilization of the left colonic flexure
	Retrieval in a specimen bag
	Safe intracorporeal anastomosis
Abdominoperineal rectum resection	
	Transection of the inferior mesenteric artery at the trunk
	Pelvic dissection
	Specimen retrieval at the perineum
	Creation of a stoma

Table 6. Evaluation of the indication for laparoscopic curative operation for colorectal carcinoma within a clinical study is justified in the following

Sigmoid carcinoma	pT1
	pT2
	pT3 (small tumor)
Abdominoperineal rectum excision	pT2
	pT3 (incipient infiltration, no lymph node bundles)
Broad-based adenoma (frequently found to be a carcinoma following histological examination) at any site	

tions we were able to justify curative laparoscopic intervention for sigmoid carcinomas pTl and pT2 or for small pT3 tumors just infiltrating the fatty tissue. However, the correct clinical staging of rectal carcinoma by coloscopic endosonography is a must (table 6).

Abdominoperineal rectal extirpation for deep situated rectal carcinoma differs fundamentally in staging from that for anterior and deep anterior rectal resection. Indications for carrying out laparoscopy for this type of operation are also favorable as the pelvic dissection is in the area of the non-tumor-carrying intestine and the actual tumor operation is approached perineally. It is important here to reach the rectum through the prescribed layers of the pelvis disengaging the mesorectum and the lateral ligaments at the same time. The laparoscopic technique demands preparation through the correct anatomical layers. If this is not performed correctly, heavy bleeding ensues. The perineal part of the operation does not differ from the conventional procedures. Positioning at the start of the descending stoma is laparoscopically more favorable as it does not interfere with the integrity of the abdominal wall. But here too there is a tight indication spectrum. Because of the relatively good results, low-risk pTl tumors are treated today with radical full wall resection. In the case of results showing advanced stage with infiltration to neighboring organs or a wide tumor infiltration into the perirectal fatty tissues as well as the lymph node system, conventional therapy should of course always be chosen.

Laparoscopic Colorectal Resections in Benign Lesions

Far less controversy exists when it comes to discussion on the possibilities of laparoscopic surgery when treating benign colorectal lesions. The following are indications for laparoscopic colorectal resection: prolapse of the rectum, sigmoid volvulus, endometriosis, Hartmann's procedure, arteriovenous malformations, diverticulitis, Crohn's disease, broad-based, raised adenomas unable to be removed endoscopically, serious obstruction, iatrogenic, traumatic and spontaneous perforations, stool incontinence, ulcerative colitis and familial polyposis as well as protective stomas in complicated anal or rectovaginal fistulas, covered rectal perforations and ischemic or radiogenic strictures [2–5, 11, 15, 16, 21, 24–34]. Due to the very low incidence rates of the individual diseases, it is difficult to obtain reliable data from single institutions regarding complication rates and long-term results. In order to obtain valid diagnostic data in a reasonable time for benign indications as well, multicentric studies as for colorectal cancer are also necessary.

Multicentric Studies

For the above-mentioned reasons, on August 1st 1995, we started a multicentric study on 'Laparoscopic colorectal surgery' in the German-speaking regions. Meanwhile, 44 clinics in Germany, Austria and Switzerland are taking part in the study (table 7). In the frame of this multicentric study all patients undergoing a laparoscopic colorectal procedure in the clinics are registered on a standard study protocol and followed up; these data are then collected centrally at the Surgical University Clinic of Erlangen. As it is an observation study, the indications for the laparoscopic colorectal operations are laid down by the individual clinics. Technical details are not dictated but simply documented. In the study framework, participants of the study are recommended to be restrictive regarding curative operations for carcinomas. However, if operations with curative intention for colorectal cancer are performed, they should be documented according to the updated questionnaire of the Working Party of the German Tumor Centers. The length

Table 7. Laparoscopic Surgery Study Group

Zentralklinikum	Chirurgische Klinik II	Augsburg
Heinz-Kalk-Klinik	Dept. für Chirurgie	Bad Kissingen
Universitätsklinikum Benjamin Franklin	Chirurgische Klinik	Berlin
Städt. Krankenhaus Zehlendorf	Chirurgische Abteilung	Berlin
Krankenhaus Buch	Allgemeinchirurgie	Berlin
Krankenhaus der Landeshauptstadt	Chirurgie	Bregenz
Evang. Diakonissenanstalt	Chirurgische Klinik	Bremen
Zentralkrankenhaus Bremen-Ost	Chirurgische Klinik	Bremen
Chirurgische Universitätsklinik		Dresden
Krankenhaus Dresden-Friedrichstadt	Chirurgische Klinik	Dresden
Städt. Krankenanstalten	Chirurgische Klinik	Esslingen
Krankenhaus Dresden-Friedrichstadt	Chirurgische Klinik	Dresden
Chirurgische Universitätsklinik		Erlangen
St.-Elisabeth-Krankenhaus	Chirurgische Klinik	Frankfurt/M.
St.-Hedwig-Hospital	Chirurgische Abteilung	Gelsenkirchen-Resse
Evang. Krankenhaus	Chirurgische Abteilung	Giessen
Kreiskrankenhaus	Allgemein- und Unfall-chirurgie	Grevenbroich
Universitätsklinikum Eppendorf	Allgemeinchirurgie	Hamburg
Allgem. Krankenhaus Ochsenzoll	Chirurgische Abteilung	Hamburg
Allgem. Krankenhaus Barmbek	Chirurgische Klinik I	Hamburg
Allgemeines Krankenhaus Altona	1. Chirurgische Abteilung	Hamburg
Krankenhaus Siloah	Chirurgische Klinik	Hannover
Klinikum Merheim	Chirurgische Universitäts-klinik	Köln
Frankenwaldklinik	Allgemeinchirurgie	Kronach
Städt. Krankenhaus	Chirurgische Klinik	Leverkusen
Chirurgische Universitätsklinik		Lübeck
Städt. Klinikum	Chirurgische Klinik	Ludwigshafen
Paracelsus-Klinik	Allgemeinchirurgie	Marl
Evang. Krankenhaus	Chirurgische Klinik	Mülheim
Klinikum Grosshadern	Chirurgische Universitäts-klinik	München
Städt. Krankenhaus Bogenhausen	Chirurgische Abteilung	München
Klinikum rechts der Isar	Chirurgische Universitäts-klinik	München
Ruppiner Klinikum GmbH	Klinik f. Allgemein- und Gefässchirurgie	Neuruppin
Ev.-Luth. Diakoniekrankenhaus	1. Chirurgische Klinik	Rotenburg a.d.W.
Klinikum Schwerin	Klinik für Chirurgie	Schwerin
Kantonsspital	Klinik für Chirurgie	St. Gallen
Klinikum Suhl	Chirurgische Klinik	Suhl
Chirurgische Universitätsklinik		Tübingen
Krankenanstalt Rudolfstiftung	1. Chirurgische Abteilung	Wien
1. Chirurgische Universitätsklinik		Wien
Wilhelminenspital	2. Chirurgische Abteilung	Wien
Städt. Krankenhaus	Chirurgie	Wismar
Bethesda Krankenhaus	Chirurgische Abteilung	Wuppertal
Chirurgische Universitätsklinik		Würzburg

of study should be about 2 years. Up to November 1st 1995, the completely filled out evaluated documentation for 62 patients is already available. This information shows that the laparoscopic colorectal operative procedures were used for very varied indications (table 8). No difficult complications occurred postoperatively in any of the patients. With the help of these studies, vast amounts of data should be available in a reasonable amount of time enabling us to make significant indications for setting laparoscopic colorectal surgery into practice.

Table 8. Laparoscopic Colorectal Study Groups Indications and operative procedures (n = 62; 1.08.1995–1.11.1995)

Resection/Extirpation (n = 46)	
Resection for cancer	n = 15 (palliative, n = 2)
Expation for cancer	n = 4
Resection for adenoma	n = 7
Resection for diverticulitis, Crohn's disease, prolaps	n = 20
Without resection (n = 16)	
Stoma	n = 5
Rectopexy	n = 7
Colon oversewing	n = 1
Hartmann's operation	n = 3

Conclusions

Till now, the indications for laparoscopic colorectal surgery have been very controversial. As, in the rule, it has only been used for selected indications, up to now only a few clinics have been able to report on large numbers of cases. Only multicentric studies can gather enough data over a short period of time to be able to set forth any conclusions concerning the indications, complications, percent changes of therapy, and long-term results. However, the experiences made until now with laparoscopic colorectal surgery influences in the spectrum of indications in such studies. This paper describes the concept of a multicentric study in the German-speaking region.

References

1 Hoffman GC, Baker JW, Fitchett CW, Vansant JH: Laparoscopic-assisted colectomy. Ann Surg 1994;6:732–743.
2 Jacobs M, Verdeja JC, Goldstein HS: Minimally invasive colon resection (laparoscopic colectomy). Surg Laparosc Endosc 1991;3: 144–150.
3 Zucker KA, Pitcher DE, Martin DT, Ford RS: Laparoscopic-assisted colon resection. Surg Endosc 1994;8:12–18.
4 Milsom JW, Lavery IC, Church JM, Stolfi VM, Fazio VW: Use of laparoscopic techniques in colorectal surgery. Dis Colon Rectum 1994;37: 215–218.
5 Phillips EH, Franklin M, Carroll BJ, Fallas MJ, Ramos R, Rosenthal D: Laparoscopic colectomy. Ann Surg 1992;6:703–707.
6 Franklin MF, Ramos R, Rosenthal D, Schüssler W: Laparoscopic colonic procedures. World J Surg 1993;17:51–56.
7 Wexner SD, Cohen SM, Johansen OB, Nogueras JJ, Jagelman BDG: Laparoscopic colorectal surgery: A prospective assessment and current perspective. Br J Surg 1993;80: 1602–1605.
8 Alexander RJT, Jaques BC, Mitchell KG: Laparoscopically assisted colectomy and wound recurrence. Lancet 1993;341:249–250.
9 Berends F, Kazerner JG, Bonjer HJ, Lange JF: Subcutaneous metastases after laparoscopic colectomy. Lancet 1994;344:58.
10 O'Rourke N, Price PM, Kelly S, Slkora K: Tumor inoculation during laparoscopy. Lancet 1993;342:388.
11 Ramos JM, Gupta S, Anthone GJ, Ortega AE, Simons J, Beart RW: Laparoscopy and colon cancer: Is the port at risk? Arch Surg 1994; 129:897–900.
12 Hermanek P, Wittekind Ch: Inwieweit sind laparoskopische Verfahren in der onkologischen Chirurgie vertretbar? Chirurg 1994;65.
13 O'Rourke NA, Head RJ: Laparoscopic surgery for colorectal cancer. Br J Surg 1993;80: 1229–1230.
14 Schlag PM, Hünerbein M, Rau B: Diagnostic and operative laparoscopy in oncology. Onkologie 1994;17:226–232.
15 Lyerty HK, Mault JR: Laparoscopic ileostomy and colostomy. Ann Surg 1994;219:317–322.
16 Fuhrmann GM, Ota DM: Laparoscopic intestinal stomas. Dis Colon Rectum 1994;37: 444–449.
17 Cohen SM, Wexner SD: Laparoscopic colorectal resection for cancer: The Cleveland Clinic Florida experience. Surg Oncol 1993;1: 35–42.
18 Tate JJT, Kwok S, Dawson JW, Lau WY, Li AKC: Prospective comparison of laparoscopic and conventional anterior resection. Br J Surg 1993;80:1396–1398.
19 Bleday R, Babineau T, Forse RA: Laparoscopic surgery for colon and rectal cancer. Semin Surg Oncol 1993;9:59–64.
20 Gray D, Lee H, Schinkert R, Beart RW Jr: Adequacy of lymphadenectomy in laparoscopic-assisted colectomy for colorectal cancer: A preliminary report. J Surg Oncol 1994;57: 8–10.
21 Franklin MW Jr, Rosental D, Norem RF: Prospective evaluation of laparoscopic colon resection versus open colon resection for adenocarcinoma: A multicenter study. Surg Endosc 1995;9:811–816.
22 Beart RW Jr: Laparoscopic colectomy: Status of the art. Dis Colon Rectum 1994;37: 547–549.
23 Köckerling F: Laparoscopic abdominoperineal excision with high transsection of the inferior mesenteric artery. Surg Oncol Clin North Am 1994;4:731–743.
24 Köckerling F, Reck T, Gastinger I: Laparoscopic abdominoperineal rectum extirpation; in Phillips EH, Rosenthal RJ (eds): Operative Strategies in Laparoscopic Surgery. Berlin, Springer, 1995, pp 242–245.
25 Köckerling F, Reck T, Gastinger I: Laparoscopic rectopexy: in Phillips EH, Rosenthal RJ (eds): Operative Strategies in Laparoscopic Surgery. Berlin, Springer, 1995, pp 246–250.
26 Decanini C, Miesom JW, Böhm B, Fazio VW: Laparoscopic oncologic abdominoperineal resection. Dis Colon Rectum 1994;37:552–558.
27 Wexner SD, Johansen OB, Nogueras JJ, Jagelman DG: Laparoscopic total abdominal colectomy: A prospective trial. Dis Colon Rectum 1992;35:651–655.
28 Schmitt SL, Cohen SM, Wexner SD, Nogueras JJ, Jagelman DG: Does laparoscopic-assisted ileal pouch anal anastomosis reduce the length of hospitalization? Int J Colorect Dis 1994;9: 134–137.
29 Cuschieri A, Shimi SM, Van der Velpen G, Banting S, Wood RAB: Laparoscopic prosthesis fixation rectopexy for complete rectal prolapse. Br J Surg 1994;81:138–139.
30 Sosa JL, Sleeman D, Puente I, McKenney MG, Hartmann R: Laparoscopic-assisted colostomy closure after Hartmann's procedure. Dis Colon Rectum 1994;37:149–152.
31 Nezhat C, Nezhat F, Ambroze W, Pennington E: Laparoscopic repair of small bowel and colon. Surg Endosc 1993;7:88–89.
32 Cuschieri A: The spectrum of laparoscopic surgery. World J Surg 1992;16:1089–1097.
33 Gorey TF, O'Connell, Waldron D, Cronin K, Kerin M, Fitzpatrick JM: Laparoscopically assisted reversal of Hartmann's procedure. Br J Surg 1993;80:109.
34 Sackier JM, Berei G, Hiatt JR, Hartunian S: Laparoscopic abdominoperineal resection of the rectum. Br J Surg 1992;79:1207–1208.

Dig Surg 1995;12:293–295

Frederick L. Greene

Department of Surgery, University of South Carolina School of Medicine, Columbia, S.C., USA

Laparoscopic versus Conventional Colon Surgery: What Are the Advantages?

Key Words
Minimal access surgery · Benefit · Outcomes

Whether one is discussing laparoscopic cholecystectomy, herniorrhaphy, management of gastroesophageal reflux disease, colectomy or a number of other intra-abdominal procedures, a reflection on the advantages of laparoscopic versus 'open' techniques is necessary in order to achieve answers to whether the laparoscopic technique is beneficial to the patient. It has been reiterated many times that the performance of a laparoscopic intra-abdominal procedure should be similar to the operation done in an 'open' manner. A well-done cholecystectomy should have the same outcome whether performed laparoscopically or through traditional means.

One of the obvious differences in the performance of laparoscopic and 'open' traditional surgical procedures is the access to the intra-abdominal cavity. A tremendous benefit of minimal access surgical procedures is that large abdominal incisions are avoided and are replaced by four to six small trocar sites that allow for the performance of the laparoscopic procedure. The reduction of abdominal wall trauma leads to less pain and more rapid recovery of the patient with return to his or her preoperative status and the necessity for less postoperative medication. Several studies have pointed to the reduction in the stress response following laparoscopic surgery and this may be secondary to the reduction in abdominal wall trauma which is realized from the laparoscopic approach [1, 2].

A second major difference between laparoscopic and conventional abdominal procedures is the utilization of pneumoperitoneum for the minimal access approach. While insufflation of carbon dioxide allows for easier manipulation of the intra-abdominal organs, there may be a downside to the creation of pneumoperitoneum because of the changes in cardiac and pulmonary physiology which occur as a consequence of developing the pneumoperitoneum [3]. In certain patients with significant coronary artery disease, close monitoring of cardiac output and identification of early arrhythmia is mandatory when pneumoperitoneum is used. Data suggest that most patients can safely be managed using a carbon dioxide-induced pneumoperitoneum. Other complications of pneumoperitoneum, such as CO_2 embolus and the creation of a pneumothorax have been described but these complications have not detracted from the overall advantage of the establishment of pneumoperitoneum. In the future, gasless techniques may become more appropriate as the technology of abdominal wall lift becomes refined [4]. Utilization of gasless techniques may also allow for the concomitant use of conventional instrumentation along with video camera techniques.

One of the far-reaching concerns that have become apparent with the use of laparoscopic techniques for cancer patients is the development of metastatic implants within the port sites in some patients [5]. These access site metas-

Frederick L. Greene, MD
Director of Surgical Oncology and Endoscopy
Department of Surgery
University of South Carolina, School of Medicine
Columbia, SC 29203 (USA)

0253–4886/95/0125–0293
$ 8.00/0

tases have been recognized following procedures for gallbladder carcinoma [6], gastric [7] and pancreatic carcinoma [8], lymphoma [9] and, more recently, management of large bowel cancer [10]. If the incidence of port-site metastases increases, the possible advantages noted above for patients with abdominal cancer may be reduced if long-term survival is jeopardized due to abdominal wall metastases. Although intra-abdominal manipulation of the tumor-bearing GI tract and retroperitoneum may be a cause of dissemination of cancer cells, the tumor biology of the cancer may actually be changed because of the creation of pneumoperitoneum. The release of intra-abdominal gas may cause a 'plume' with shedding of cells in the port sites. These cells may then be trapped by fibrin plugs if appropriate hemostasis is not maintained within the trocar site. In addition, the withdrawal of tumor-bearing tissue through either trocar sites or small abdominal incisions may cause tracking of cancer cells which promote abdominal wall growth. It is obvious that surgeons who perform minimal access oncologic techniques must learn to handle tissue gently and must protect the abdominal wall much as has been advocated over decades when bacterial contamination is likely. If the occurrence of abdominal wall metastases continues to escalate, the overall advantages of minimal access surgery for the patient with abdominal cancer may be overshadowed.

One of the little known, but metabolically important secondary events of the creation of a pneumoperitoneum is the increase in endogenous arginine vasopressin [11]. The effect of this active hormone is to cause constriction of the vascular bed which may be important as more intra-abdominal anastomoses of the gastrointestinal tract are performed through laparoscopic means. In addition, portal blood flow and renal blood flow are diminished as the intra-abdominal pressure of the pneumoperitoneum increases. This may be a consequence of increased vasopressin outpouring as a direct response to increased intra-abdominal pressure. A greater concern is noted by realizing that vasopressin also enhances overall clotting of blood by increasing the procoagulants such as factor VIII and von Willebrands factor [12]. The importance of this change in coagulation is realized, especially in a cancer patient who, because of the effect of the tumor, may have an already hypercoagulable state created. Although outcome studies have not defined increased deep venous thrombosis in cancer patients, there are reports of clotting in patients undergoing laparoscopic cholecystectomy [13]. Because of the effect of pneumoperitoneum on the levels of arginine vasopressin, the surgeon must utilize protective mechanisms against abnormal clotting. Techniques, such as use of alternating compression devices on the legs and subcutaneous heparin, are important to reduce the possible consequences of hypercoagulation during minimal access techniques.

The overall advantage of minimal access abdominal procedures is seen in the enhancement of quality of life of patients who need abdominal surgical procedures. This quality of life improvement is secondary to reduced pain, reduced length of hospital stay, faster return of gastrointestinal function and alimentation, reduced need for postoperative analgesia, and, most importantly, return to preoperative levels of activity and enjoyment of family following the performance of a laparoscopic surgical procedure. If laparoscopic surgical techniques can be done safely and efficiently with reduction of overall cost to society, the advantages of these new techniques clearly outweigh operations performed using traditional abdominal incisions.

Economic Benefit

Economic considerations of medical care continue to be of paramount interest throughout the world and no matter what method of health care payment is used. In the United States the bill for health care was USD 280 billion in 1980 and is estimated to be close to one trillion dollars in 1995. It is obvious that the cost of medical care cannot be looked upon as only the individual cost in the operating room or as a result of hospitalization but must be judged in terms of the global effect of medical care on patient outcome and the ability to return to work in a timely manner.

Several cost analyses of laparoscopic surgery and, specifically, laparoscopic cholecystectomy, have been undertaken throughout the world [14–16]. Although the overall cost of laparoscopic cholecystectomy is made up of many factors, only 19–25% of the total cost is a result of operating room expense. The major impact of laparoscopic surgery on global cost is judged on the ability to return the patient to the work force in a timely manner. In addition, Ure et al. [14] form Germany have shown that by shortening the hospital stay and reducing the time of inability to work, at least 33% of the total cost of medical care may be attributed to these areas. It is obvious that through the use of minimal access techniques, the large portion of global medical care cost may be reduced when hospital stay is reduced to 1 day and patients return to work in just a few days after their laparoscopic cholecystectomy. Although the debate continues regarding the overall cost of disposable versus reusable equipments, studies have shown that with the increasing prevalence of laparoscopic cholecystectomy in a hospital, the differences in overall cost between disposable and reusable instruments may be equalized [17]. It is clear that some procedures, such as laparoscopic herniorrhaphy, may drive up the total cost of a procedure based on the equipment used without realizing an overall benefit when judged against conventional outpatient herniorrhaphy performed by an anterior approach.

The surgeon must play an important role in the determination of cost in the hospital and the operating room. Attention to efficiency and the mandatory use of specialized teams to perform laparoscopic surgery will assure continued reduction of operating room time which will result in a significant cost saving. Although, initially, the performance of laparoscopic surgical procedures may be lenghty when compared to 'open' surgery, as surgeons become more proficient in the application of minimal access techniques, the overall operating time will be diminished. As was suggested by Eiseman and Borlase [18], cost-effectiveness in clinical practice should be evaluated as follows: (1) is there a cost reduction; (2) is there an effective improvement in health care; (3) does the cost reduction produce an equal or better outcome, and (4) is there an additional benefit that justifies the additional cost? It is obvious that when one considers laparoscopic techniques, the answer to these important questions is certainly in the affirmative.

References

1 Bessler M, Whelan RL, Halverson A, et al: Is immune function better preserved after laparoscopic versus open colon resection? Surg Endosc 1994;8:881–883.

2 Allendorf JD, Bessler M, Kayton ML, et al: Increased tumor establishment and growth after laparotomy vs. laparoscopy in murine model. Arch Surg 1995;130:649–653.

3 Dorsay DA, Greene FL, Baysinger CL: Hemodynamic changes during laparoscopic cholecystectomy monitored with transesophageal echocardiography (TEE). Surg Endosc 1995;9:128–134.

4 Smith RS, Organ CH Jr: Gasless Laparoscopy with Conventional Instruments. The Next Phase in Minimally Invasive Surgery. San Francisco, Norman, 1993.

5 Nduka CC, Monsom JRT, Menzies N, et al: Abdominal wall metastases following laparoscopy. Br J Surg 1994;81:648.

6 Drouard F, Delamarre J, Capron JP: Cutaneous seeding of gallbladder cancer after laparoscopic cholecystectomy. N Engl J Med 1991;325:1316.

7 Cava A: Subcutaneous metastasis following laparoscopy in gastric adenocarcinoma. Eur J Surg Oncol 1990;16:63–67.

8 Siriwardena A, Samarji WN: Cutaneous tumor seeding from a previously undiagnosed pancreatic carcinoma after laparoscopic cholecystectomy. Ann R Coll Surg Eng 1993;75:199–200.

9 Aractingi S, Morolleau JP, Daniel MT, et al: Localisations sous-cutanées de lymphome de Burkitt aux points de pénétrations d'un cœlioscope. Ann Derm Vénéréol 1993;120:796–797.

10 Fusco MA, Paluzzi MW: Abdominal wall recurrence after laparoscopic colectomy for adenocarcinoma of the colon. Dis Colon Rectum 1993;36:858–861.

11 Punnonen R, Viinamaki O: Release of arginine vasopressin related to increase in intra-abdominal pressure. Lancet 1982;i:175–176.

12 Nussey SS, Bevan DH, Ang V, et al: Effects of arginine vasopressin (AVP) infusions on circulating concentrations of platelet AVP, factor VIII:C and von Willebrand factor. Thromb Haemost 1986;55:34–36.

13 Caprini JA, Arcelus JI, Laubach M, et al: Postoperative hypercoagulability and deep-vein thrombosis after laparoscopic cholecystectomy. Surg Endosc 1995;9:304–309.

14 Ure BM, Lefering R, Troidl H: Costs of laparoscopic cholecystectomy. Surg Endosc 1995;9:401–406.

15 MacFadyen BV, Lenz S: The economic considerations in laparoscopic surgery. Surg Endosc 1994;8:748–752.

16 Wenner J, Graffner H, Lindell G: A financial analysis of laparoscopic and open cholecystectomy. Surg Endosc 1995;9:702–705.

17 Reichert M: Laparoscopic instruments. AORN J 1993;57:637–655.

18 Eiseman B, Borlase BC: Measurement of cost effectiveness; in Eiseman B, L Stahlgren (eds): Cost-Effective Surgical Practice. Philadelphia, Saunders, pp 1–5.

Dig Surg 1995;12:296–301

P. Buchmann
D. Christen

Department of Surgery, Stadtspital Waid, Zurich, Switzerland

Pro Laparoscopic Surgery for Colorectal Cancer

Key Words
Minimal invasive surgery · Colorectal cancer · Cytology · Safety

In May 1993, we started with laparoscopically assisted colorectal surgery after extensive experience in laparoscopic cholecystectomy, appendicectomy, adhesiotomy and fundoplication. Up to March 1995, we carried out laparoscopic colorectal operations in 137 patients. Eighteen (13%) were converted to open surgery. Forty-nine patients (6 = 12% conversion rate) suffered from benign disease, 22 (1) from a rectal prolapse including 13 (0) with additional sigmoid resection, and 66 (11 = 16%) from large bowel cancer. After completing this series we feel that five topics concerning laparoscopically assisted colorectal carcinoma surgery have to be discussed: (1) education; (2) cost; (3) confort; (4) technique, and (5) safety.

Education

A few years ago, the attitude towards education in laparoscopic surgery was: 'First learn the technique of open surgery and then turn to laparoscopic procedures.' Evaluation of laparoscopic cholecystectomy has taught us a different lesson. Today it is almost impossible to start with open cholecystectomy because most patients demand minimal invasive surgery. Only the more difficult cases are subjected to laparotomy. Even the most conservative hardliners now accept that endoscopic operation has to be learned first and admit that the anatomy is better seen and easier to understand on the screen.

Training can begin with working on a pelvitrainer to become familiar with basics. The value of the animal laboratory is questioned, especially with respect to animal protection and costs. It is believed that the lab should be used in the evaluation of new procedures but not to increase skill. Training is most effective in the technique of manipulating the camera and suction, together with that of using the various other instruments.

At the moment we have the situation where teachers switch to becoming pupils again. Experienced surgeons have to learn do deal with new instruments and a new technology. The inevitable learning curve has to be minimalized by proceeding from easier operations, e.g. cholecystectomy or appendicectomy, to more demanding procedures like adhesiotomy. For colonic resections we prefer to begin with right hemicolectomy, and then to proceed to sigmoid and low anterior resections. It would also be desirable to do operations for benign lesions first, but unfortunately only a few patients present with such pathology in the terminal ileum or ascending colon, whilst resection for diverticulitis can be much more difficult than a T_1 or T_2 carcinoma. Therefore, we are convinced that effective tutoring must be established before hospitals start with minimal invasive colonic surgery.

Cost

The costs of laparoscopic surgery are of great concern to hospital authorities. The high expense of the equipment is followed by continuing outlay on disposable instruments, especially staplers and clip applicators. With increasing

We thank Mr. G.D. Oates, Birmingham, UK, for the careful editing.

Prof. P. Buchmann
Department of Surgery
Stadtspital Waid
Tièchestrasse 99
CH–8037 Zürich (Switzerland)

0253–4886/95/0125–0296
$ 8.00/0

Table 1. Cost

	Laparoscopic	Open
Theatre	+	–
Postoperative		
Pain killers	–	+
Infusions	–	+
Hospitalisation	(–)	=
Time off work	–	+
Political economy	?	?

Table 2. Comfort

	Laparoscopic	Open
Pain	–	+
Hospital stay	(–)	=
Time for recovery	–	+
Cosmetics	+	–
Summary	+	–

Table 3. Technique

Operation	Laparoscopic	Open
Incision	3×stab incisions 1×short incision	1×long incision
Intraabdominal	clips	ligations/clips
Anastomosis		
Right (left) hemicolectomy	hand sewing	hand sewing
Sigmoid-rectum	double stapling	stapling (double)

practice such costs can be reduced, mainly in laparoscopically assisted resections (e.g. clipping the inferior mesenteric artery instead of using an endostapler). However, open surgery will always be cheaper in the theatre (table 1). The difference is probably not even compensated by the reduced requirement for analgesics and infusions resulting from the lesser degree of pain and the earlier return of bowel function.

Hospital stay may initially be the same, but with more confidence in the new method it should decrease, resulting in lower expenses for hospitalisation. Because of the very small incisions, recovery from surgery is much faster and earlier return to work is possible after a minimal invasive procedure [1, 2]. It seems logical that the economic benefit must be significant but no data are available either for laparoscopic or for open surgery.

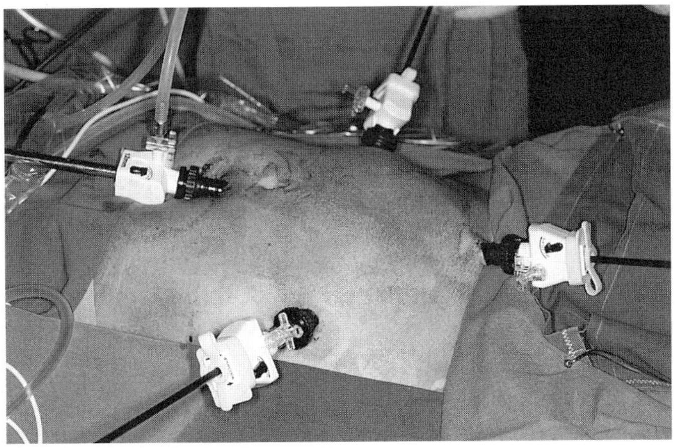

Fig. 1. Positioning of the 4 trocars.

The need for expensive disposable instruments increases from laparoscopically assisted right hemicolectomy with the possibility of hand-sewn anastomosis to sigmoid and low anterior resection where dissection of the rectum alone usually requires at least two endostaplers for the double-stapling technique.

Comfort

There is general agreement concerning the confort of laparoscopic surgery (table 2). The small incisions result in less pain and a satisfactory cosmetic outcome of the operations. Earlier discharge from hospital and a shorter period of recovery are further advantages. However, there are not valid arguments if the extent of resection in cancer surgery is less radical than it would be in open surgery.

Technique

No compromise can be allowed in the performance of laparoscopic surgery. Operative steps are identical in both laparoscopically assisted and open resections. Only some technical details may be different (e.g. ligation versus clipping) (table 3). The access to the abdomen for all colonic resections is by 4 trocars (between umbilicus and xyphoid, right and left side as well as suprasymphysic) (fig. 1) or a midline incision, respectively. Maximal intraabdominal pressure is 12 mm Hg and we use a 3-chip camera with a 25° or 30° angeled optic.

Safety

When an established operation is replaced by a new technique the safety of the new procedure must be of major concern (table 4). Intraoperatively, the view is much better in laparoscopic than in open surgery because of the fourfold magnification of the scope but the ability to palpate is missing. On the other hand, the tumor is never touched even if located very low in the pelvis since good camera vision can be achieved even in the rectorectal-presacral space.

Some recent publications indicate that there may be less impairment of immunologic defense mechanisms by minimal invasive procedures, e.g. delayed-type hypersensitivity reaction was the same pre- and postoperatively after a laparoscopic operation in Sprague-Dawley rats but decreased after open surgery [3], or hypochlorus acid production by neutrophils was unchanged after minimal invasive bowel resections compared with a disruption following conventional interventions in man [4]. These findings are of extraordinary interest for the future assessment of laparoscopic cancer surgery because one could speculate that an intact immune mechanism early after removal of a carcinoma might be beneficial in respect to tumor cell killing.

Up to now we have no information about long-term follow-up after laparoscopically assisted colon carcinoma surgery, although we anticipate achieving the same survival rates as in open procedures. The problem of port-site metastases is not yet resolved and will be dealt with below. Since the risk of provoking local tumor spread in minimal invasive cancer surgery is still an unanswered question, informed consent by patients after detailed discussion is mandatory. Centers performing this type of surgery should enter all cases into a prospective controlled study to guarantee quality control and follow-up.

Table 4. Safety

	Laparoscopic	Open
Intraoperative		
View	+	–
Palpation	–	+
Postoperative		
Immunology	+	–
Follow-up	?	well known
Risks	?	well known

Table 5. Prospective controlled study comparing laparoscopically assisted cancer surgery (n = 45) with matched open resections (n = 44): tumor staging and grading

	Laparoscopic	Open
TNM		
pN0	30	23
pN1–2	10	16
M1	5	5
Grading		
G1	3	3
G2	36	37
G3	6	3

Table 6. Prospective controlled study comparing laparoscopically assisted cancer surgery (n = 45) with matched open resections (n = 44): length of formalin fixed specimens (cm)

Operation	n	Laparoscopic	Open
Right hemicolectomy	11/11	21.0	24.0
Left hemicolectomy	2/2	28.5	21.0
Rectosigmoid resection	18/18	19.0	18.0
Low anterior resection	10/10	19.0	19.5
Proctectomy	4/3	23.0	28.0

Our Results

We have analyzed our initial 45 patients with carcinoma operated on by a laparoscopically assisted technique up to December 1994 against matched patients with identical open resections. The results were presented at the annual meeting of the German Society of Surgeons in Berlin 1995 [5].

All patients who gave informed consent were operated endoscopically, excluding those with an extremely extensive tumor requiring a large incision to bring out the specimen and those tumors exhibiting wide infiltration into neighboring organs or the abdominal wall. Patients in risk category ASA 5 were also excluded.

The average age of the patients was 68 (29–88) years and of the matched open-resected patients 70 (40–92 years). In both groups there were 22 females and 23 (22) males (1 man treated by laparoscopic proctectomy was not matchable). We compared 11 right hemicolectomies, 2 left hemicolectomies, 18 rectosigmoid resections, 10 low anterior resections, and 4 (3) proctectomies. Tumor classification and grading are listed in table 5. In the minimal invasive group pNo were most frequent but grading demonstrated almost identical status of tumor differentiation.

The results are summarized in tables 6–8. The length of resected bowel measured by the pathologist on the formalin-fixed specimen was comparable (table 6). The same was

Table 7. Prospective controlled study comparing laparoscopically assisted cancer surgery (n = 45) with matched open resections (n = 44): number of lymph nodes

Operation	n	Laparoscopic	Open
Right hemicolectomy	11/11	13.0	13.0
Left hemicolectomy	2/2	12.5	9.5
Rectosigmoid resection	18/18	16.0	10.0
Low anterior resection	10/10	13.0	11.0
Proctectomy	4/3	10.0	12.0

Table 8. Prospective controlled study comparing laparoscopically assisted cancer surgery (n = 45) with matched open resections (n = 44): number of blood transfusions during the whole hospitalisation

Operation	n	Laparoscopic	Open
Right hemicolectomy	11/11	2.0	2.0
Left hemicolectomy	2/2	2.0	2.0
Rectosigmoid resection	18/18	2.0	3.0
Low anterior resection	10/10	6.5	4.0
Proctectomy	4/3	5.0	9.0

Table 9. Prospective controlled study comparing laparoscopically assisted cancer surgery (n = 45) with matched open resections (n = 44): postoperative complications

	Laparoscopic	Open
Rebleeding	4 (1)	1
Wound infection	2 (1)	4 (1)
Dehiscence of anastomosis	3 (2)	2 (1)
Pneumonia	3	1
Urinary infection	–	1
Deep vein thrombosis	–	–
Cardiopulmonary decompensation	–	3
Port-site metastasis	1	–
Death	1	2

( ) = With reoperation.

true for the number of lymph nodes (table 7). The volumes of blood transfusions were recorded during the whole period of hospital stay, and were increased only in the low anterior resection (table 8) because of bleeding complications in the first third of the laparoscopically operated group (table 9). We concluded from these data that laparoscopically assisted resection of colorectal carcinoma is as radical as conventional open operation and the need to replace blood is comparable.

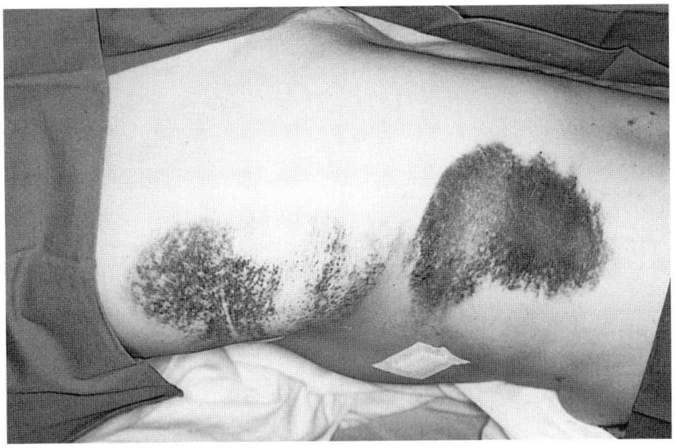

Fig. 2. Hematoma of the lateral abdominal wall after laparoscopically assisted rectosigmoid resection.

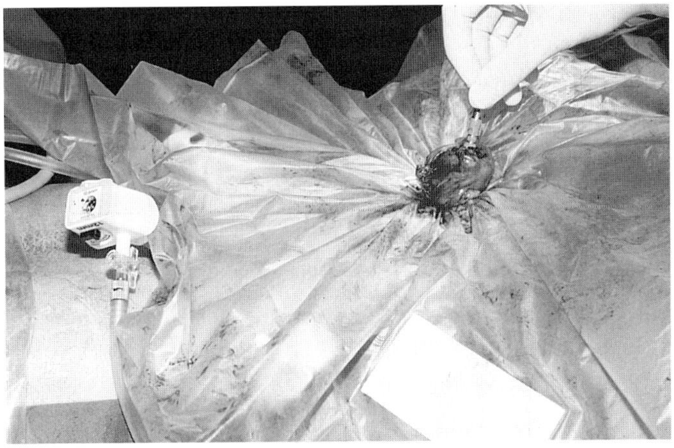

Fig. 3. Wound protector

Risks of Laparoscopically Assisted Cancer Surgery

Three main risks are noted: bleeding, wound contamination during bringing out the specimen and implantation of tumor into the wound as reflected by port-site metastases (table 9). The problem of bleeding is already mentioned above. We noted three extensive hematomas in both groups of patients, and in one we had to reoperate because of an overlooked laceration of a pelvic vessel caused by the mandrel of the circular stapler (fig. 2). With more experience we should be able to reduce bleeding complications. No wound infections have developed since we employed a wound protector during the procedure of pulling out the bowel (fig. 3).

Table 10. Port-side metastases and theories of pathogenesis

	Laparoscopic	Open
Squeezing the tumor	–	+
Local ischemia	trocar	retractor
Capillary flow	trocar	drains
	drains (wound protector)	(wound protector)
Whirling of tumor cells	?	–

Anastomotic dehiscence was noted after a right hemicolectomy in a poor-risk patient and in two low anterior resections after preoperative irradiation with 46 Gy. The single death in the laparoscopic group was due to a myocardial infarction on the day before planned discharge. During follow-up of 1–20 months, we detected one port-site metastasis 9 months after right hemicolectomy for a pT_4 pN_1 M_1 carcinoma. The trocar has been located within 2 cm of tumor infiltration into the abdominal wall and a drain was led through the same tract. No locoregional recurrence was noted in the same period.

Port-site metastasis after laparoscopic cancer surgery is a widely and sometimes emotionally discussed subject. The many case reports and small series in the literature give an inadequate picture of the risk. In a prospective trial of 208 laparoscopic colorectal cancer resections 3 (1.4%) port-site metastases were found. Two of these 3 patients suffered from peritoneal carcinomatosis [6].

In a retrospective analysis over a period of 25 years and 5,273 patients with open resections 48 (0.9%) soft tissue metastases were detected [7]. Resectable implanted tumors had a 5 years' survival of 30% but metastases apart from incisions or drain tracts had bad prognosis and usually reflected a progressive carcinoma.

Some theories of the pathogenesis of port-site metastases are listed (table 10). Since in minimal invasive surgery touching the tumor is never necessary, the squeezing hypothesis can be dismissed. Local ischemia and a capillary flow exist in both laparoscopic and open surgery. During endoscopic operation a trocar moves in and out even when fixed with a screw thread. In our series to date this has not been responsible for any postoperative complications. We known too little of the effect of capillary flow possibly bearing tumor cells and local ischemia to formulate a statement. However, from open surgery we know that metastases may occur at drain sites. Therefore, it seems logical to suspect a similar mechanism at the port-site. The hypothesis of whirling the tumor cells by the gas insufflation is controversial. It is questioned if tumor cells are freed during a laparoscopic procedure and if they survive in CO_2.

We started a prospective study of abdominal wash out at the beginning of the operation, after ligation of the major vessels, the end of cancer mobilisation and finally at the end of pneumoperitoneum, using 200 ml of saline each time followed by a cytologic search for tumor cells. Thirty-nine patients were studies (table 11). Positive cytology was found in 3 patients and in 1 severe dysplasia (table 12). The patient with peritoneal carcinomatosis died after 1 month without metastases and the 3–8 months follow-up of the other 3 patients has been uneventful, though too short for any reliable conclusions.

Answers to the Initial Questions and Summary

Education. A new approach to teaching is needed. The use of models (e.g. pelvitrainer) helps us to get accustomed to the two-dimensional view. Young surgeons will have less difficulties than traditionally trained operators since they start with a new technique from the very beginning. Experienced surgeons should accept experts in minimal invasive surgery as their tutors in order to reduce their learning curve.

Cost. At first sight laparoscopically assisted colorectal surgery seems to be more expensive than open resection. However, judgement must be made in a wider context taking into consideration all aspects, and especially the 'political economy' (table 1). This topic needs urgent evaluation for both laparoscopic and open procedures if we are to demonstrate a benefit from minimal invasive surgery. Politicians and hospital authorities must seek compensation for the high intraoperative costs in order to reduce financial deficits in public hospitals.

Comfort. The superiority of endoscopic surgery is indisputable (table 2).

Technique. Specialized instruments for minimal invasive surgery have been developed and further progress is continuing. Technical problems concerning intraabdominal procedures have been solved. Any compromises in laparoscopic operations are forbidden.

Safety. The radical extent of resection is equal in both techniques (tables 6, 7). With increasing experience complication rates can be reduced to or below those of open procedures (table 9). The same is true for the need for blood transfusions (table 8).

The development of port-site metastases has to be reviewed carefully. They tend to grow in patients with an advanced carcinoma at the time of operation, especially when peritoneal carcinomatosis is present (table 11). We do not know whether we should exclude extensive cancers from

Table 11. Results of cytologic examination of washout (n = 39)

	Laparoscopic		Open	
	negative	positive	negative	positive
pT_1 pN_1	2	–	–	–
pT_2 pN_{0-1}	2	(1)	1	–
pT_3 pN_{0-3}	15	–	8	1
pT_4 pN_{0-3}	–	–	4	–
M_1 pT_{3-4}	–	1	2	–
Peritoneal carcinomatosis	–	–	1	1
	19	2	16	2

Table 12. Positive washout cytology in colorectal cancer (n = 4/39)

TNM	Time of sampling			
	beginning	ligation	mobilisation	end
pT_2 pN_0	–	–	stong reactive alterations	–
pT_4 pN_1	+	–	–	–
Peritoneal carcinomatosis	+	+	+	–
pT_3 pN_0	analysis of whole amount			

minimal invasive surgery or accept the risk of implantation of metastases. Further studies must be carried out to clarify this question. We are very eager to know the late outcome of any patient with a positive wash-out cytology (table 12).

A possible advantage of minimal invasive surgery is the absence of impairment of immune status. However, its influence on recurrence rates and survival is not yet predictable.

Conclusion

The pros of laparoscopic surgery for colorectal cancer are concentrated so far on perioperative advantages (comfort, recovery, time off work). Risks and possible benefits in respect of recurrence rates and survival are not yet known, although, the radical extent of surgery is identical in endoscopic and open techniques. Minimal invasive surgery for malignant colorectal disease must be done as part of a prospective controlled trial.

References

1 Vanek VW, Bourguet CC: The cost of laparoscopic versus open cholecystectomy in a community hospital. Surg Endosc 1995;9: 314–323.

2 Tucker JG, Ambroze WL, Orangio GR, Duncan TD, Mason EM, Lucas GW: Laparoscopically assisted bowel surgery. Surg Endosc 1995;9:297–300.

3 Trokel MJ, Bessler M, Treat MR, Whelan RL, Nowygrod R: Preservation of immune response after laparoscopy. Surg Endosc 1994;8: 1385–1388.

4 Carey PD, Wakefield CH, Thayeb A, Monson JRT, Darzi A, Guillon PJ: Effects of minimally invasive surgery on hypochlorous acid production by neutrophils. Br J Surg 1994;81: 557–560.

5 Buchmann P, Christen D, Bischofberger U, Flury R: Die laparoskopische Chirurgie des Kolonkarzinomes. Ein Vergleich mit der offenen Technik. Langenbeck Arch Chir, in press.

6 Ramos JM, Gupta S, Anthone GJ, Ortega AE, Simons AJ, Beart RW: Laparoscopy and colon cancer. Arch Surg 1994;129:897–899.

7 Hohenberger W: Weichteilmetastasen: Referat 112. Kongr Deutsch Ges Chir 1995, in preparation.

Dig Surg 1995;12:302–306

Ch.A. Seiler

Department of Visceral and Transplantation Surgery, University of Berne, Inselspital, Berne, Switzerland

Laparoscopic Resection for Colorectal Cancer: A Safe Way to Cure Cancer?

Key Words
Laparoscopic resection · Colorectal cancer · Savety

Introduction

Praxagoras was said to have performed the first colonic decompression in the history of colonic surgery in 400 BC. In 1826 the Frenchman Lisfranc, surgeon under Napoleon, was the first person to remove a cancerous tumor from the rectum, essentially made by means of a transanal operation. Reybard of Lyon, France, however, was the first surgeon to perform a successful resection of the sigmoid colon with primary anastomosis in 1833 through a formal laparotomy, thus introducing colorectal surgery into medicine [1–4]. Since then colorectal surgery has developed into one of the main disciplines in surgery, based on an impressive background of development, experience and academic sciences. 158 years after the first open colectomy and only some few years ago (1991) several small series of laparoscopic colonic resections were published by Jacobs and others, introducing a new technique and thus opening a new chapter of colonic surgery [5, 6]. This new endeavor faces us now with a lot of new uanswered questions.

Oncologic Background and Epidemiology

Colorectal cancer is the second most frequent cause of male and the third cause of female cancer death, secondary only to lung and breast cancer. The cancer death rate for colorectal cancer is 20–30 per 100,000 people worldwide, despite the fact that more than 50% of colorectal cancer nowadays is curable with 'open' surgical techniques [7, 8]. Thus, colorectal cancer still represents one of the most important healthcare problems in medicine which has a tremendous impact on healthcare politics as well as on healthcare economics. Any changes in treatment modality may therefore greatly influence not only healthcare but more importantly may have a significant influence on survival and cure of colorectal cancer.

Laparoscopic Surgery

When Mouret, on March 1st 1987, performed the first laparoscopic cholecystectomy, no one would have imaged the chain reaction of acceptance and spread which followed thereafter. Within a few years, this minimal invasive technique has become the gold standard of removing the gallbladder. Soon other indications for this new technique were introduced such as appendectomy, antireflux surgery (fundoplication) and colonic surgery. Based on the progressive experience the advantages of the laparoscopic technique became more and more evident, i.e. less pain due to less abdominal wall trauma, shorter hospital stay and earlier return to work. However, since the first attempts were made attacking malignant disease by the laroscope, the question of

Ch.A. Seiler, MD
University of Bern
Department of Visceral and Transplantation Surgery
Inselspital
CH–3010 Bern (Switzerland)

0253–4886/95/0125–0302
$ 8.00/0

cosmetics, postoperative comfort and reduction in hospital stay is no longer relevant but the absolute vital issue in this situation is the chance of cure of cancer and the likelihood of recurrence of cancer disease, compared to the standard of open surgical technique. In converting to malignant disease laparoscopic surgery has left the safe lonely island of benign disease and has now to face and withstand the big stormy ocean of cancer surgery.

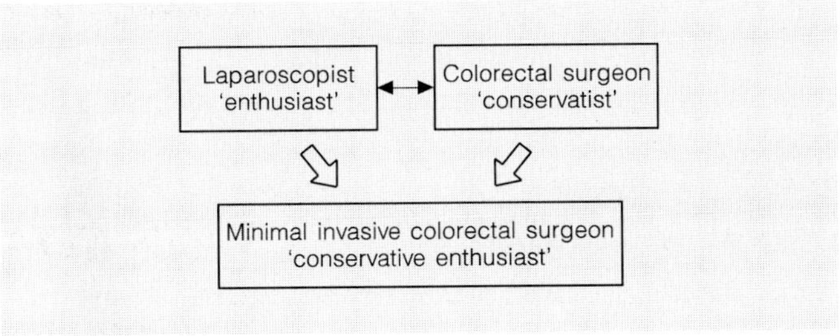

Fig. 1. The dilemma of 'experience' in laparoscopic colorectal surgery.

Laparoscopic Surgery in Colorectal Disease

The surgical speciality of colorectal surgery is common, especially in the United States, where many surgeons perform only colorectal operations. These colorectal surgeons concentrate a tremendous load of knowledge and background information on colorectal disease, not only regarding technical skills but even more in terms of therapeutic strategies to achieve optimal long-term cure with minimal side effects. However, correct colorectal surgery is not easily accomplished by the laparoscopic technique. Since laparoscopic colorectal surgery is technically extremely demanding, this technique cannot be learned within a few days in a training course. On the other hand, there are some very skilled laparoscopic surgeons who have had the opportunity to build up their laparoscopic technical abilities in a variety of different operations with increasing technical skills. These kind of surgeons have the optimal technical background to perform the demanding operations of colorectal resections. But does this laparoscopic surgeon possess the extensive background knowledge on colorectal surgery, especially specifically regarding treatment for colorectal cancer compared to his conventional/open surgical college? This brings us to the dilemma between the conservative colorectal surgeon representing the knowledge of more than 150 years of colorectal surgery and on the other hand the laparoscopic surgeon who may lack this knowledge. The final aim of the American Society of Colorectal Surgeons and the Society of American Gastrointestinal and Endoscopic Surgeons was to create guidelines on how to convert colorectal surgeons into minimal invasive colorectal surgeons. These guidelines have been published in 1991, at the same time as the first reports of laparoscopic colon resection appeared [9, 10]. However, the question of how to convert a laparoscopic enthusiast into a knowledgeable and reliable/serious colorectal surgeon is still open (fig. 1). Reports on laparoscopic colorectal resections usually differ substantially from the documentation reported by colorectal surgeons. Thus, the comparison of both techniques with regards to (long-term) outcome is not possible. Only until recently was there increasing information from the newly generated group of 'minimal invasive colorectal surgeons' which allowed comparable data retrieval [11, 12]; although these two societies have underlined the importance that 'laparoscopic colorectal surgery should be undertaken only in a setting in which proper prospective data retrieval occurs'. Five years later the demands for 'statistically valid scientific data should replace personal opinion' and 'patients should no longer be sacrificed to achieve a triumph of technology over common sense' [12] still exist.

Morbidity of the Laparoscopic Approach in Colorectal Surgery

Contrary to open cholecystectomy where laparotomy and laparotomy closure are the major part of the operation regarding duration and surgical trauma, laparotomy in colorectal surgery is only a minor trauma compared to the major dissection of several abdominal quadrants often combined with extensive pelvic dissection. Thus, only a modest reduction in minor postoperative morbidity is expected to be achieved by the laparoscopic approach. However, the important question is whether a new technology is able to reduce major morbidity and failure. In colorectal surgery this means reducing the incidence of *anastomotic leak.* There is no reason to think that the anastomotic leak rate will be reduced by the laparoscopic approach with its rigid access (ports) to the bowel (to be anatomosed) and its impaired facilities to safety test the anastomosis for leaks during the operation. *Injury* to vital structures like the ureter, arteries or the intestine are imminent, especially in obese patients. Mobilization of the greater omentum of the transverse colon causes a particular difficulty for the laparoscopic surgeon. There are risks of damage to the middle colic artery, stomach and duodenum. The use of diathermy remains a potential hazard to this structure [11, 13]. There is increased concern about the raising incidence of *thromboembolic complications* despite prophylaxis againts deep-vein thrombosis. The combination of a prolonged pneumoperitoneum and the possible reduction of deep venous bloodflow, combined with surgical trauma close to the compressed (pneumoperitoneum) iliac vessels and the almost unavoidable cave compression generated by the Loyd-Davies position, is a major concern causing morbidity and mortality [13]. However, the Achilles heel of laparoscopic colonic surgery is the *specimen retrieval* which almost always makes a laparotomy unavoidable. The major advantage of minimal invasive surgery is lost by performing a sort of open access. The length of a laparotomy, however, is less important with regards to morbidity than the fact that there is in fact a laparotomy. Therefore, simply reducing the size of the laparotomy wound will lead only to a very modest reduction in postoperative morbidity if at all.

The overall morbidity of laparoscopic surgery for colorectal disease is unlikely to be reduced compared to an open technique. One of the larger series of laparoscopic colorectal surgery for colorectal disease reports a minor morbidity rate of 24% and a major morbidity of 29% [14]. Consequently, laparoscopic procedures in colorectal surgery must first prove to be safe before they can become a standard of care. A high complication rate will quickly offset the claimed advantages of cost effectiveness by reduced hospital stay after laparoscopic surgery, when patients suffer a higher complication rate compared to open surgery.

Laparoscopy and the Principals of Cancer Surgery

The safety of the laparoscopic approach to malignant disease is a point of great concern and dispute. Since colon cancer is curable by open surgery in up to 50% of the cases the possible benefits of the laparoscopic approach in terms of cosmetics, reduced pain scores, shorter hospital stay, and accelerated return to normal activity must be balanced against the possibility of reduced cure rates.

The laparoscopic approach perioperatively allows only a visual inspection of the tumor and is thus affecting the quality of *tumor staging*. However, accurate perioperative localization of the lesion and of possible secondaries has a tremendous influence on the treatment plan (extension of resection, resection margins, etc.) and on the long-term results lacking palpation. Many of the colonic tumors are not readily visible at laproscopy. This requires an intraoperative colonoscopy which adds time to an already lengthy operative procedure or the patient has to undergo a preoperative colonoscopy with injection of India ink by puncturing the lesion [15].

To follow the rules of the *no-touch technique*, most surgeons will use a hand or a swab to distract the colon during mobilization in open surgery which is effective and atraumatic. This contrasts considerably with the laparoscopic procedure in which Babcock forceps must be used. These forceps are traumatic and relatively inefficient; the more efficient they are, the more traumatic they are. The laparoscopic surgeon is totally dependent on gravity for packing away the small bowel during extensive colonic dissection. The 'natural' retraction of the small bowel is limited by a critical angle of the Trendelenburg position and the retracting instruments are generally out of camera view during dissection with its possibility of damaging the intestine. For final mobilization of the tumor, it is, however, technically unavoidable not to touch the lesion with the traumatic Babcock forceps lacking other instruments.

The concern of *tumor cell shedding* and subsequent implantation is highly conceivable [16–18]. In laparoscopic surgery the cytocydal washout, especially of the proximal end of the gut, is virtually impossible and hardly mentioned in the laparoscopic literature [11].

Although some authors present a comparable amount of *lymph nodes*, resected with the specimen in open and laparoscopic technique [14, 19], this is a crude criteria to judge the adequacy of resection. There are important differences from institution to institution regarding the amount of resected lymph nodes. Furthermore, it can be well influenced by many other variables like the use of preoperative treatment strategies (radiotherapy). Finally, the sensitivity of this analysis is very dependent on the carefulness and skills of the pathologist. The laparoscopic approach has clearly defined technical limits compared to the open surgical approach, especially in the region of the lesser sack where it is virtually impossible to resect all lymph nodes according to the oncological principles of tumor surgery by the laparoscopic approach.

Finally, the specimen protection and *specimen retrieval* implies increased manipulation and the possibility of tumor shedding. In the rare cases where the specimen can be removed transanally, unphysiogical dilatation of the anal sphincter is caused. The bigger the specimen, the more difficult it is to remove from the abdomen. Morcellation of the specimen intraabdominally in order to deliver the specimen through a small incision is unacceptable in malignancies. The extraction of the tumor through a small-port laparotomy brings the cancer in direct contact with the peritoneum and the abdominal wall. By putting the tumor into a bag before the retrieval makes it safe for the retrieval itself but causes an additional risk of tumor cell shedding during intraabdominal manipulation during placement of the tumor into the sack.

Port-Site Metastasis

Port-site metastasis after laparoscopic colorectal surgery for cure of malignancy was first reported in 1993 [20]. This bizarre complication was absolutely new, not only to laparoscopic surgeons, but to open surgeons as well since wound-site recurrence after standard laparotomy is unrecognized. None of the major textbooks of colorectal surgery mention this complication. In the world literature there is only one single serious report mentioned in which 11 patients from 1,603 cases had recurrence associated with the laparotomy incision or the drainage tube site, showing an incidence of 0.7% of wound-site recurrences [12, 21]. In contrast, 33 port-site recurrences have been published within a 2-year time span, from 1993 to 1995. The incidence of this bizarre complication is 6.3% (1.5–21%) and the interval between operation and occurrence of the port-site metastasis was 7.2 (3–26) months after surgery [12]. Whether the almost 10 times increased incidence of port-site recurrences compared to wound-site recurrences in open surgery is realistic, cannot yet be answered comprehensively. But the number of reported cases undoubtedly represents only the tip of the iceberg due to the delay from occurence to publication. The scary fact is that one third of the published port site recurrences was derived from Dukes-A and Dukes-B cancer stages and is not exclusive to advanced lesions! Several other questions remain open regarding port-site recurrences. Why do port-site recurrences not all recur at the port of specimen retrieval? Why does the recurrence after conversion to open surgery (4.5–41%) [11] not occur at the laparotomy wound but at the port-site? Why do port-site recurrences occur in all cancer stages, not only in widespread disease? And why do we make the same observations not only in colorectal cancer but in gynecological malignancy [22] as well? Are these phenomena due to insufficient surgical technique? What is the influence of the pneumoperitoneum on this phenomenon? Is this due to reduced perfusion or changed local immunological reaction? Or is it a new unrecognized aspect of tumor biological behavior? All these questions need to be answered before the laparoscopic technique is used to remove malignancies with curative intention.

Prime Aim of Colorectal Cancer Surgery

In contrast to laparoscopic surgery for benign disease where patient comfort, cosmetics and hospital stay are important issues, the prime aims of treatment for malignant disease are widely different. The prime aims of colorectal cancer surgery are to improve *long-term cure,* to reduce *loco-regional recurrences,* to cause *fewer stomas,* to avoid *autonomic nerve damage* and to improve overall quality of life in *reducing long-term morbidity.* In a review of more than 120 publications of laparoscopic colorectal surgery none of them could by far prove to reach these goals [11]. Until the present, there is no *prospective randomized trial* available comparing open and laparoscopic techniques in a comparable setting, although thousands of laparoscopic colectomies have been performed. The ethical question still remains whether laparoscopic surgery for colorectal cancer is not trading cure and long-term survival for improved short-term recovery. At present, it is difficult to advocate laparoscopic surgery for cure of colorectal cancer since many very vital questions have not yet been answered. Therefore, laparoscopic surgery for colorectal cancer should no longer be performed outside of a *prospective randomized trial* analyzing long-term survival rates regarding tumor classification and staging. The claim of pioneering in this field of surgery is no longer valid since many years. To perform a surgical procedure for cure of cancer with an unproven outcome outside the setting of a carefully controlled data retrieval may consequently end in sacrificing more potentially curable patients than is ethically acceptable.

References

1 Cormann ML: Colon and Rectal Surgery. Philadelphia, Lippincott, 1993, pp 514–517, 596–601.
2 Amussat J-Z: Mémoire sur la possibilité d'établir un anus artificiel dans la région lombaire sans pénétrer dans le péritoine. Dis Colon Rectum 1983;26:483.
3 Lisfranc J: Mémoire sur l'excision de la partie inférieure du rectum devenue carcinomateuse. Dis Colon Rectum 1983;26:694.
4 Reybard JF: Mémoire sur une tumeur cancéreuse affectant l'iliaque du colon: Ablation de la tumeur et de l'intestin; réunion directe et immédiate des deux bouts de cet organe. Bull Acad Méd, Paris 1843–44;9:1031.
5 Jacobs M, Verdeja JC, Goldstein HS: Minimal invasive colon resection (laparoscopic colectomy). Surg Laparosc Endosc 1991;1: 144–150.
6 Corbitt JD Jr: Preliminary experience with laparoscopic-guided colectomy. Surg Laparosc Endosc 1992;2:79–81.
7 Cormann ML: Colon and Rectal Surgery. Philadelphia, Lippincott, 1993, pp 566–569, 643–646.
8 American Cancer Society: Ca – A Cancer Journal for Clinicians 1989;39:3–39.
9 Society of American Gastrointestinal Endoscopic Surgeons: Granting of privileges for laparoscopic general surgery. Am J Surg 1991; 161:324–325.
10 American Society of Colon and Rectal Surgeons: Policy statement. Dis Colon Rectum 1992;35:5A.
11 Monson JRT, Hill ADK, Darzi A: Laparoscopic colonic surgery. Br J Surg 1995;82: 150–157.
12 Wexner SD, Cohen SM: Port site metastases after laparoscopic colorectal surgery for cure of malignancy. Br J Surg 1995;82:295–298.
13 Guillou PJ, Darzi A, Monson JRT: Experience with laparoscopic colorectal surgery for malignant disease. Surg Oncol 1993;2(suppl 1): 43–49.
14 Falk PM, Beart RW Jr, Wexner SD, et al: Laparoscopic colectomy: A critical appraisal. Dis Colon Rectum 1993;36:28–34.
15 Hill ADK, Banwell PD, Darzi A: Laparoscopic colonic surgery: The unseen lesion. Minim Invas Ther 1993;2:171–172.
16 Umpleby HC, Fermor B, Symes MO, Williamson RCN: Viability of exfoliated colorectal carcinoma cells. Br J Surg 1984;71: 659–663.
17 Fermor B, Umpleby HC, Lever JV, Symes MO, Williamson RCN: Proliferative and metastatic potential of exfoliated colorectal cancer cells. J Natl Cancer Inst 1986;76: 347–349.
18 Skipper D, Jeffrey MJ, Cooper AJ, Alexander P, Taylor I: Enhanced growth of tumour cells in healing colonic anastomoses and laparotomy wounds. Int J Colorectal Dis 1989;4:172–177.
19 Monson JRT, Darzi A, Carey PD, Guillou PJ: Prospective evaluation of laparoscopic-assisted colectomy in an unselected group of patients. Lancet 1992;340:831–833.
20 O'Rouke N, Price PM, Kelly S, Sikora K: Tumour inoculation during laparoscopy (letter). Lancet 1993;342:368.
21 Hughes ES, McDermott FT, Poliglase AI, Johnson WR: Tumor recurrence in the abdominal wall scar after large bowel cancer surgery. Dis Colon Rectum 1983;26:571–572.
22 Gleeson NC, Nicosia SV, Mark JE, et al: Abdominal wall metastases from ovarian cancer after laparoscopy. Am J Obstet Gynecol 1993; 169:522–523.

Author Index Vol. 12, No. 5, 1995

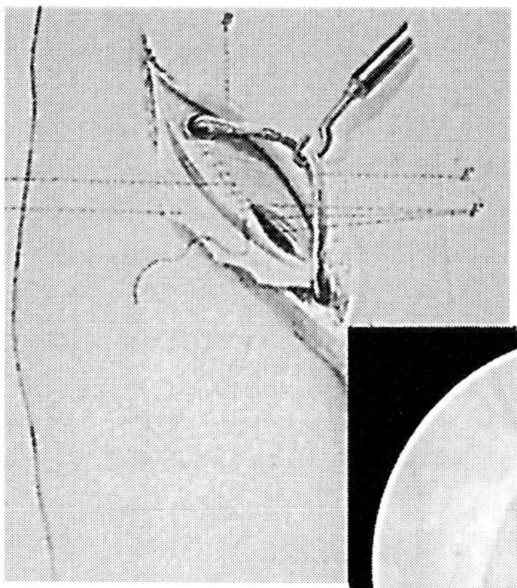

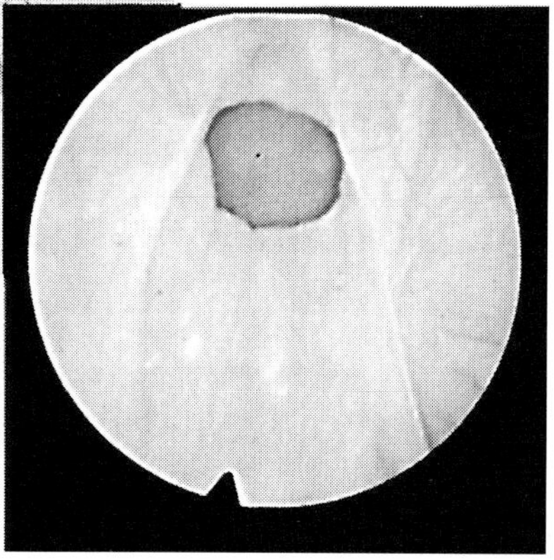